DISSENTING
DIAGNOSIS

DISSENTING
DIAGNOSIS

DR ARUN
GADRE

DR ABHAY
SHUKLA

Foreword by Keshav Desiraju

PENGUIN BOOKS

An imprint of Penguin Random House

PENGUIN BOOKS

USA | Canada | UK | Ireland | Australia
New Zealand | India | South Africa | China | Singapore

Penguin Books is part of the Penguin Random House group of companies
whose addresses can be found at global.penguinrandomhouse.com

Published by Penguin Random House India Pvt. Ltd
4th Floor, Capital Tower 1, MG Road,
Gurugram 122 002, Haryana, India

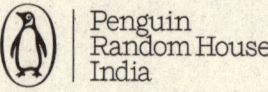

Penguin
Random House
India

First published by Random House India 2016
Published in Penguin Books by Penguin Random House India 2018

ISBN 9788184007015

Typeset in Adobe Garamond Pro by Manipal Digital Systems, Manipal

Printed at Repro India Limited

Based on a study by SATHI, Pune

(Support for Advocacy and Training to Health Initiatives)

Contents

Contents

Foreword

There are several large questions in public health in India today to which the answers are ambiguous at best: Is the state responsible for providing health care? What is meant by the right to health? Do citizens need legal protection to access health care? Do we, or do we not, in India, subscribe to Universal Health Care? Who pays for health care? Who is responsible for the regulation of health care and services, and for the professional conduct of doctors? This remarkable book, compiled by Arun Gadre and Abhay Shukla based on interviews with seventy-eight doctors, attempts to look at some of these questions. I use the word remarkable advisedly; in the closed and competitive world of private medical care it could not have been easy to get practising doctors to introspect on their profession, and to admit to the cynicism and bad faith which prevails.

The world of private medical care, which is believed to account for 80 per cent of all health care transactions in India, is spread over a wide range, from the large corporate hospitals of the metro cities to smaller hospitals and nursing homes and individual practitioners. There is near consensus amongst the doctors interviewed that patients are often put through unnecessary expenditures, that medical practice is largely unregulated, that self-regulation has not succeeded and that invidious links exist between drug manufacturers, pharmacies and middlemen of every sort, including even autorickshaw drivers. It is not, of course, the case that these ills exist only in private practice. It is not also the case that private practice alone lends itself to perversion.

The point quite simply is that the practice of the profession has itself suffered. Traditionally, doctors have always enjoyed great social prestige and the gratitude of their patients, but this has not spread across the board to higher personal or professional standards, or to the highest ethical standards.

The authors have correctly observed that a reform of the system must come with an overall increase in government investment in health care and medical education, with a reform of the current regulatory mechanisms, including the councils and a much greater public ownership of the sector. India is clearly not in a situation where private investment or private insurance can take on the burden of primary care; for the conceivable future, governments, both at the centre and in the states, must increase investment, not least in medical and nursing education, towards the universally accepted norm of 3 per cent of GDP. Whether by design or by accident, the privatization of medical education is rapid. Of the approximately 425 medical colleges functioning today, well over half are private, accounting for 48 per cent of the approximately 53,235 seats at the MBBS level. Newly trained doctors, who have paid handsomely for their training are, almost by definition, unavailable for modestly paying jobs in the public sector. Unless state governments invest in medical and nursing education, especially in the underserved states, we can expect little by way of a strengthened primary health care system.

All doctors must read this book, and health policymakers, and all those interested in the future of public health in India.

Chennai   Keshav Desiraju
13 December 2015

Introduction

Health and health care should be treated as basic rights for every human being. These rights are an inalienable part of the Right to Life, which is one of the fundamental rights enshrined in the Constitution of India. This perspective has guided us and our work with the health sector non-governmental organization (NGO), SATHI for over one-and-a-half decades. During this journey, one of our most important observations has been that while the majority of patients turn to private medical services for a variety of reasons, there is large-scale dissatisfaction regarding the quality of services, unaffordable costs of care, and unnecessary procedures and surgeries often conducted in private medical facilities. It is clear that the laws regulating private medical services are very weak or non-existent, while their implementation is so perfunctory that, effectively, these services are completely unregulated. Though the private medical sector is a behemoth that dominates the entire health care scenario, since it is unregulated and lacks any standardization, this giant has feet of clay. Given this context, the central government passed the 'Clinical Establishment Act' in 2010 to regulate private medical services across the country.

However, instead of welcoming standards to regulate their profession, most associations of private doctors bitterly opposed this Act. While some of this opposition is directed at certain deficiencies and lacunae in the Act, the basic stand of most doctors' associations can be summed up as follows: 'We private doctors are doing an excellent job of regulating ourselves. All is well, though there may be a few rare exceptions. So there is no need for society and the state to regulate doctors.'

We decided to study this issue to get to the truth of the situation. We turned to the dwindling but significant number of 'rational' doctors, those whom we knew are so, even today, trying to conduct their practice in an ethical manner. The first author of this book, Dr Arun Gadre, has been in private practice as a gynaecologist for more than twenty years, and knew, from his personal experience, of doctors who practised rationally and ethically. Though the terms 'rational' or 'ethical' are laden with subjectivity, if we define a 'rational doctor' as one who treats patients as advised in textbooks, and define the term 'ethical doctor' as one who advises only the indicated investigations, procedures or surgery according to established, evidence-based guidelines (such as those found in standard textbooks), then the *kind* of medical practitioner we are referring to becomes clear. Practising doctors always have an accurate idea of the nature of their colleagues' practices. Cross references, as well as the grapevine, are sound methods of establishing this. For this survey, Dr Arun Gadre posed questions to the doctors about their experiences: In the current state of their profession, was everything working well or were there deeper secrets hidden? If everything was not working well, what were the reasons? These questions became the starting point, based on which, with support from the network of SATHI and Jan Swasthya Abhiyan, we took the exploration forward and contacted a larger circle of doctors across the country. We were pleasantly surprised to find that though few in number, such rational voices within the medical profession were present in every place we searched for them.

This book contains the thoughts and reflections of such rational[1] doctors: their critical introspections, their 'dissenting diagnosis', which runs counter to complacency about the state of medical practice displayed by mainstream associations of private doctors. These doctors are courageously holding up a mirror to the profession. Their 'voices of conscience' are full of righteous anger, yet they also reflect a sense of helplessness at the sorry state of this once 'noble profession'.

We should not lose sight of the wider factors that have led to this situation. Since the 1990s, like all sectors of Indian society, the health care sector has been swept up in the whirlwind of globalization, liberalization and privatization. How did it come to pass that a well-intentioned, service-oriented profession was transformed into a market-driven commodity, and then into a corporate-led, profiteering industry? It was as if most doctors—preoccupied as they were with their own individual practices—were unable to comprehend this sweeping process. In just a few decades, the entire context of the private medical sector was transformed. Pharmaceutical companies, insurance companies, corporate hospitals, medical equipment companies, private medical colleges, multinational vaccine manufacturers—all these powerful actors related to the private medical sector have been united in their drive for expanding profits, and they have ensured that health care becomes more and more of a commodity in the marketplace, their shiny goods (of sometimes doubtful benefit) being available only to those who can afford their escalating costs.

Not only did the social logic of the medical profession fall by the wayside, even the logic of rational medical practice was increasingly blown away by the all-encompassing imperative of profit. Medicine dealing with the suffering and death of human beings has always possessed an element of social logic. The doctor has to prioritize the patient's well-being first, not the doctor's own self-interest. But those who were grounded in the idea of service have felt the ground swept away from under their feet, their traditions of 'keep the patient foremost' rapidly buried under the ruthless logic of 'keep profits foremost'.

In this context, the reflections of these seventy-eight rationally practising doctors from various parts of the country may sound like the swan song of a species on the verge of extinction. But the concerns that are being raised are not restricted to doctors alone. These anguished voices are now finding wider resonance, in the form of deeply felt, popular dissatisfaction and simmering anger, regarding practices in the private health care sector. Sporadic but growing attacks on private hospitals are the regrettable but inevitable consequence of a problem that is now too large to be pushed under the carpet.

Unfortunately, many governments today are withdrawing from their responsibility to provide quality health services to people and are resorting instead to 'public-private partnerships' (PPPs). Eager votaries of such PPPs and state-supported health insurance schemes would have us believe that the state should hand over large-scale public funds to the private medical sector, based on the uncritical assumption that private providers will provide good quality health care to the population. In this context, these scathing reflections on the private medical sector from within the medical profession provide us with a healthy counterview. These observations give us a glimpse of what we might expect if the state decides to hand over responsibility for providing health care on a large-scale to unregulated, profit-driven private agencies, without effective regulation and rationalization.

The backdrop to this situation is that in the past few decades, under the influence of privatization- and liberalization-oriented policies, public health services have been left underfunded. They are also often prone to corruption and not adequately responsive to ordinary patients. Not only does the middle class keep well away, but in many places even the poor are abandoning public health services and turning to private services. The chilling reality is that in order to cover the costs of using private medical services, the poor are forced to sell their homes and land. According to the World Health Organization, in the past few years approximately 3.5 per cent of the population per annum (amounting to nearly four crore people) have been pushed below the poverty line in India, just on account of expenditures incurred by them on expensive private medical services. They are forced to resort to these services since they cannot access good quality public health services.

Many doctors' associations do not examine this frightening reality with any seriousness. The stand of some of these organizations is to deny that there is any problem at all. The stand of a doctor's association has consistently been that while there may be a few black sheep, the majority of doctors are conducting their medical practices ethically and properly. How do doctors, who conduct their practices honestly, regard private medical services that have become the dominant providers of health care? To what extent do these doctors themselves feel that the current situation is serious and dangerous? What are the solutions that can, in the opinion of these doctors, be devised to tackle this situation at a systemic level? What, in short, do they—indeed any doctors dissatisfied with the degeneration of the system—think about it all?

The public at large is probably unaware of the helplessness felt by such doctors who are deeply troubled about the entire scenario. The public sees the insistent and self-congratulatory posture of certain doctors' associations, or newspaper reports about attacks on hospitals, and the cases that are brought before the consumer courts, as well as sensational media reports on deaths in private hospitals caused by negligence. If, for instance, a healthy thirty-year-old dies during a simple operation, the doctor's negligence may not be a factor. But the perception of society is that many doctors today exploit patients, putting them through investigations, surgeries and procedures which are not needed. Even a suspicion of negligence can lead to a public reaction which can all too easily flare up into violence, which, however deplorable, has to be understood in the context in which such extreme reactions arise. There has been a decline of transparency in the medical sector, and the overall position of many doctors and their associations has been one of complicit silence or active support of the guilty.

Against this background, there are two advantages in bringing into the public domain the voices of rationally practising, ethical doctors.

Firstly, we can examine the claim that 'there are only a few doctors who are engaged in unethical practices, but the entire medical profession is being blamed'. This dubious assertion can best be critically dissected by practising doctors themselves.

Secondly, this will help alert doctors and their associations, the general public, the government and public health bureaucracy, consumer organizations, ordinary patients, the media, and researchers working on issues of health to the urgent need for change. When doctors themselves expose the stark reality of the private medical sector, there will no longer be any grounds for doubt about the magnitude of the problem.

Methodology and Analysis of the Study

The doctors who have been interviewed for this book include both well-known doctors as well as less-widely-known doctors from Maharashtra, Chhattisgarh, Bangalore, Delhi, Kolkata and Chennai. This includes doctors practising in megacities like Mumbai, Bangalore, Kolkata and Delhi; in cities like Pune, Nasik and Sangli; in small towns, and even doctors practising in villages. We are grateful to Dr Vijay Ajgaonkar, diabetes specialist from Mumbai; a surgeon and activist from a megacity, who has played an important role in highlighting unethical medical practices; Dr Sanjay Gupte, former president of the Federation of Obstetric and Gynaecological Societies of India (FOGSI), Pune; Dr H.V. Sardesai; senior physician in Pune, Dr Arjun Rajgopalan; senior general surgeon in Chennai; and Dr Sanjib Mukhopadhyay, senior gynaecologist in Kolkata.

We made a detailed transcript of all interviews, in which we picked up the essence of what each doctor was saying, and have formed the categories, which you are now about to read. The purpose of making such categories is to help the reader sharply understand the critical dimensions of each situation. With these categories, the reader will be able to understand exactly the point that the doctors want to make through their examples. Of course, it is very rarely that doctors have spoken exclusively on only one particular subject. But when an example is placed in a particular category, it means that the example becomes focused on that particular issue.

Table 1: Details of 78 Doctors Interviewed

Distribution based on work in private practice, not-for-profit or public/academic institution	
Private practitioners	66
Public/academic institute	7
Not-for-profit/charity hospitals	5

Geographical distribution	
Cities	
Bangalore	9
Chennai	7
Delhi	11
Kolkata	7
Mumbai	5
Nasik	5
Pune	17
Medium- and small-sized towns	
Small- and medium-sized towns in Maharashtra	16
Small town in Chhattisgarh	1

Distribution based on qualification	
Anaesthetist	3
Cardiologist	2
Cardiothoracic surgeon	1
Dentist	1
ENT surgeon	1
Gastroenterologist	3
Gynaecologist	9
Interventionist	1

Distribution based on qualification	
MBBS (General practitioner)	9
Nephrologist	4
Ophthalmologist	4
Orthopaedic surgeon	1
Paediatrician	6
Pathologist	3
Public health expert	4
General physician	6
Psychiatrist	1
Radiologist	1
Skin specialist	3
General surgeon	10
Urologist	1
BAMS	2
BHMS	2

Distribution by level of specialization	
Super-specialist	13
Specialist	52
General practitioner	13

Whether they own a hospital	
Yes	10
No	68

Whether attached to a corporate/multi-specialty hospital	
Yes	27
No	51

Permission given to reveal personal identity	
Yes	37
No	41

Years of experience of practice	
Less than ten years	2
Ten to twenty years	7
Twenty to thirty years	16
More than thirty years	53

How These Doctors Were Selected

The doctors to be interviewed were identified through personal contacts, and then through a further chain of doctor contacts.[2] This is not a representative sample, and we make no claim that the views of these seventy-eight doctors reflect the views of the entire medical profession. In fact, it is an oft expressed opinion that it is relatively difficult to locate ethically practising doctors, who may be regarded as 'exceptions' within their profession, hence this specific method had to be adopted.

The initial circle of doctors was from among those whom the first author, Dr Arun Gadre, knew personally, and who were known to be practising ethically. Other doctors, especially outside Maharashtra, were located through the contacts of ethical doctors, or contacts of colleagues in SATHI, who had personally experienced these doctors' ethical and rational practice.

Dr Arun Gadre interviewed this set of doctors—regarding whom there was some evidence that they were ethical and rational in their practice—who were willing to be interviewed, and place their views in the public domain. One by one, the seventy-eight doctors were interviewed all over India, of which sixty-six had private practices and twelve did not.

The dozen doctors who did not have private practices had close knowledge of the nature of the private medical sector. These included Dr Vandana Prasad, paediatrician and former member of the National Commission for Protection of Child Rights (2012–13); Dr L.R. Murmu, additional professor of surgery at the renowned public hospital, All Indian Institute of Medical Sciences (AIIMS) in New Delhi; Dr Chandrakant Pandav, head of the department, Centre for Community Medicine, AIIMS; and Dr Punyabrata Goon of Shramajibi Swasthya Udyog from Kolkata. These twelve doctors relate intensively with the private medical sector, and either treat patients coming from the private sector or have studied the private sector in some form. Many private doctors often send patients with complicated illnesses or terminal diseases to a premier government hospital like AIIMS as a dumping ground. Apart from that, poor people come to such hospitals when private doctors recommend a course of treatment they cannot afford. For these reasons, doctors working in hospitals like AIIMS have significant knowledge of the workings of the private medical sector.

Each of these doctors gave written consent to record their oral, face-to-face interviews. In certain cases, due to lack of time for an oral interview, selected doctors sent in written answers to our questions. An effort has been made to reproduce responsibly their words exactly as they were expressed. The recordings of the interviews have been carefully preserved as proof of the accuracy of the transcriptions.

Thirty-seven doctors who participated in the study gave permission to use their names, and their names have therefore been mentioned in this book. Both authors have been in private practice themselves and know the pitfalls. For instance, there is the ever-present anxiety that even without a mistake on their part, a patient under their care may die or develop serious complications. In such a situation, there is no effective mechanism that can help them, while there is a tendency among doctors in the private sector to point fingers at other doctors. There are increasing incidences of attacks on private doctors and hence individually practising doctors feel quite vulnerable. The incidences can happen in public hospitals too, but the mighty arm of the government is available to back up doctors in public hospitals. In the private set-up, the doctor has to fight on his or her own. Secondly, no doctor in private practice ever wants a scuffle on the premises as his or her reputation is at stake. Hence many honest doctors in private practice are apprehensive about alienating their colleagues while exposing malpractices in the private medical sector. Therefore, the names and locations of those doctors in the sample have been kept confidential at their request.

The interviews given by these doctors who are currently engaged in private practice, all point towards an important and serious reality. This reality is the deplorable decline in ethical standards in private medical services, and also the highly commercialized form that such practice has acquired. But even more than this, they make it clear that in our midst there is still a group of doctors, albeit a small one, who, just like most patients, feel suffocated by this gross commercialization and are deeply disturbed by the unethical practices that are rampant. Barring a few very senior, well-established doctors, the majority of these young and middle-aged doctors are engaged in a tough day-to-day struggle to avoid compromise and keep themselves out of the jaws of unethical, commercially-driven practice, which has become the dominant norm.

It is a genuine fear among many that such doctors may, soon, like some endangered species, become extinct. If we are to avoid this, then society must rapidly identify structures and mechanisms that would ensure protection of rational practice and provide safeguards against unethical practices.

All doctors were asked nine common questions:

1. Are you satisfied with the private medical sector as it functions today?
2. If not satisfied, then tell us the areas in which standards have gone down and problems have arisen.
3. From your experience, can you give us some examples of medical malpractice?

4. Give some examples from your own experience of irrational practices which cause harm to patients.

5. Can you give some example of inflated rates being charged for medical services?

6. What is the impact of the growth of corporate and multi-speciality hospitals on the medical profession?

7. What is the impact that insurance has on the functioning of hospitals?

8. What is the influence of pharmaceutical companies on the functioning of hospitals?

9. What suggestions do you have to improve the current situation?

Dr Arun Gadre personally contacted all these doctors and conducted the interviews. He drew on his twenty years of private practice as a gynaecologist in a rural area. All doctors participated fearlessly in the interviews and shared their observations freely. Thirty-seven doctors have also given written permission to use their names.

As we outline the conclusions, opinions and insights gained from these interviews, we first present the complete interview of Dr Vijay Ajgaonkar from Mumbai—a leading diabetes specialist, professor, and a well-established figure in medical circles. His interview reflects many of the themes that emerge from interviews with the other doctors. The emphasis varies according to their experience of medical practice, specialization, geographical location and qualifications.

In Part One of this book, these rational doctors speak on the wide range of symptoms that emerge from the deep underlying malaise of the health sector in India today. However, we have tried not just to describe the symptoms and outline the diagnosis, but have also attempted to put forth a range of possible solutions to this situation in the second part of the book. The reader may or may not agree with all the solutions, but writing this book was certainly a challenge. Our colleagues at SATHI, Dr Anant Phadke and Dr Nilangi Sardeshpande provided valuable assistance. The chapter on Universal Health Care (UHC) is based on a booklet for which the primary drafting was done by our former colleague, Dr Amita Pitre. And this book would not have been possible without the support of Penguin Random House India, and particularly the guidance and positive encouragement of the editor-in-chief, literary publishing, Meru Gokhale. We are sincerely grateful to all of them.

Finally, we would like to express the hope that this book will be of some use, in terms of being a 'wake-up call' for society in general and doctors in particular, about the need to ensure social regulation and transparency in the private medical sector. In a sense, this book is a 'public hearing' on the private medical sector, conducted by a section of private doctors themselves. We hope that the searing testimonies will help awaken the general public, citizens' groups, social movements, and political representatives to the urgent need for regulation in the private medical sector in India. We hope that with social pressure and political attention, this sector, that has remained largely unregulated until now, will be subjected to participatory and social regulation in the interests of ordinary patients, as well as rational health care professionals. That would be the best response we could give to the anguished voices of ethical doctors that are reflected in this book.

Part One:

Diagnosing the Malady

Chapter 1

Complete Interview:

Dr Vijay Ajgaonkar, senior diabetologist, Mumbai

Question: There is a growing demand from society for effective regulation of the private medical sector. What is your opinion on this subject?

Dr Ajgaonkar: There are no two ways about it. Regulation of medical practice is of course necessary because we have collectively not been able to maintain the ethics of our profession and we have let it become a business! That is the state of affairs today.

Why should doctors work? To serve the people. Now any person who says to himself, 'This "service" stuff is too much, I can't do it,' should not come to study medicine. The nature of our profession earlier was service-oriented. What were the medicines that were used in earlier times? They were often placebos . . . Let me explain about placebos to your readers. They are tablets without any effective ingredient in them—but they are given as treatment anyway, so that the patient feels better, since they feel that have received some kind of care. People used to feel better even with those placebos. The reason was because there was a relationship of trust between doctor and patient.

Now under the onslaught of technology, we have lost our clinical sense. Do you understand the seriousness? We doctors used to rely on our skill to pick up signs. As we grew older we used to develop that marvellous sixth sense. Now we have lost it thanks to our dependence on investigations. Often, an illness has psychological origins. I myself have often seen cases where just a few minutes of sympathetic conversation with a patient has resulted in a dramatic decrease in blood sugar levels. But see what is happening—American fads or I would rather say commercial fads are now getting established here. Like doing full body investigations routinely without any indication. Just fling a set of statistics in the patient's face. 'The prognosis is . . . 97 per cent mortality!' So is it really like this? First, ninety-seven patients will die, and only after that will three be saved? No, it's not like that, is it? Are doctors some kind of gods? No? Then they should boost that patient's morale. A patient's will to live can be strong . . . and if the doctor builds up his morale and these [factors] come together, people live on, casting aside all kinds of gloomy prognoses. I have seen such cases myself. We can't say which patient fits into this pattern. Medicines alone do not help; the doctor-patient relationship is tremendously important. We seem to have forgotten these principles nowadays. What we treat are figures for blood pressure and blood sugar, X-rays, MRIs and CT Scans. We don't treat human beings. Even during our medical training, we dissect parts of the body. . . we never look at a person as a whole.

Now everything in medicine has become mechanical. Doctors too have changed. I will tell you about doctors in earlier days. Dr Modi was forty years my senior. But he used to come to Chembur to examine my patients. He charged just Rs 50 and what did he tell the patient? 'The medicines given by Dr Ajgaonkar are all appropriate and I am not going to change even one.' Dr Wadia would make a diagnosis just based on the patient's detailed case history, and would decide the course of treatment after examining the patient. It was only rarely that he would order investigations.

Now our greed has increased to the extent that when a patient of one consultant goes to another consultant, the second one prescribes the same medicine, but merely changes the brand to show that he is doing something different. And it is true that this profession has now become a completely commercial business.

If you look at the issue objectively, it is not our role to make money by taking advantage of another person's illness. But that is exactly what is happening. They put terminally ill seventy- to eighty-year-olds on ventilators, keeping the hospital meter running by unnecessarily using the ICU and ventilator. Come on, just let the patient go home. Let him die in peace at home amidst his family members. In the ICU there are tubes in the mouth and nose . . . the patient can't speak even if he wishes to.

Of course, when the patient is young, and the disease is reversible . . . certainly you should use the ventilator. But what is the point in pushing forward for a short while an old man's death—that too while you ruin him financially and increase his sufferings?

Doctors angrily question why there is no regulation on builders and property developers. In the first place, we are not builders but doctors. We deal with issues of life and death! That is not the case with the builders and developers. And then, if we ourselves start behaving like builders, people will also treat us as such. Have we ever imposed any self-discipline on ourselves? No. If we ourselves do not keep ourselves well dressed and start dancing in the nude, why would other people tolerate our behaviour? They will take steps to cover us decently. How can we then complain, 'You are interfering with our work?' How dare we complain? You tell me, do we have any right to do that?

And what a terrible state we have reached! The pharmaceutical companies have tried to entice us with big temptations, and we have fallen prey to them. Simply because it's free . . . just because pharmaceutical companies give [doctors] free alcohol, senior, eminent doctors get drunk in public programmes . . . when one sees this, one is disgusted, ashamed. Drink if you want. But go to your room and drink, not in public with the free liquor given by drug companies. Once you are in the pharmaceutical companies' debt, then you have to prescribe unnecessary medicines produced by them.

And as to pharmaceutical companies . . . yes, some new molecules are useful. But what about the price? Just see . . . insulin was available at Rs 30 or so per dose, now it costs around Rs 150. How is that? The research costs on the medicine have been recovered—should the medicine become cheaper or more expensive over time? No medicine ever becomes cheaper. How is that? I for one never attend pharmaceutical company-sponsored meetings, and if I do go, I never eat anything other than a salad.

Often, largely useless medicines—medicines that have no additional benefit compared to existing cheaper variants—are palmed off. And even if any defects come up in the post-marketing survey . . . the companies don't disclose this information and continue to market the same medicines.

And now huge corporate hospitals and multi-speciality hospitals are growing. These hospitals put pressure on all the doctors linked to the hospital, and on their full-time doctor employees. They demand that they must send a certain quantum of business to the labs and the radiologists. There is no doubt that this practice has become commonplace. Unnecessary investigations are then forced upon the patients. The unfortunate patients are trapped. They keep running from one big hospital to the other. This is what is going on today.

KEM Hospital, Nair Hospital, JJ Hospital[1] are all teaching hospitals, and procedures like angioplasty are performed there too. If well supported, these teaching hospitals can easily do better than all these corporate and multi-speciality hospitals. In that case, we should increase the facilities in these government hospitals. But our elected representatives . . . have now become self-representatives. The facilities in public hospitals are not improved. Government hospitals are being ruined through deliberate neglect. Just as MTNL is being killed off so that private mobile companies can profit . . . the government hospitals are being neglected so that corporate hospitals may benefit.

Now see . . . the radiology unit and lab have been outsourced by two of the largest public hospitals in Mumbai. Why was this done? The same reason—to promote the private sector. How can the poor afford this? One does not understand. Why would private hospitals do anything for free? Of course they avoid giving free services; there is no doubt about it.

The history of these corporate hospitals and the influence they wield is frightening. My father established an association for a particular medical condition. It set up a hospital for the poor in a small building in Mahim, Mumbai. Members of the association were charged concessional rates for all services. When I was working there, my OPD would be the most crowded; people would queue up from 5 a.m. But then the hospital was taken over by a corporate hospital. Since it was a hospital run by a trust, they could not buy it directly. So then they took over the management of the association. They paid the membership fees of our lower-level staff to enrol them as members, and got a majority of votes in favour of corporate takeover. For the general body meeting of the association, the lower-level staff was brought there in buses, and subsequently they were taken to an expensive hotel for lunch.

The doctors were also no different from the administration. Many of them would sign without even examining the patient and prepare a bill. They would do this with inpatients and patients in the operation theatre. Such doctors, too, happily joined the corporate bandwagon and also voted for it. And thus the corporate lobby finally took over the hospital management, and built a separate twelve-storey, air-conditioned hospital building. Hospitalization there for just two days would cost around Rs 50,000. I could not bear to see this, and resigned. Then they, too, were unable to manage the hospital—it has now been taken over by Fortis.

It is not just corporate hospitals, what is going on all around is unspeakable; violations occur everywhere.

I will give you an example from Pune. A judge was about to be appointed to a higher post and as part of the process went to a well-known doctor appointed by the government for this purpose. The doctor declared the judge unfit, saying that his blood pressure was high. The judge was angry. He checked his blood pressure elsewhere: it was normal! So he went back and confronted the doctor. The doctor told him without embarrassment, 'Will you be able to pay me X amount of money?'

The judge shot back, 'Tomorrow I will be presiding as a judge. Should I change my judgement because one of the parties in a case comes to me with money? I will go to Mumbai and get a genuine certificate from another doctor. I will try not just once but ten times, and I will of course never give any money. And once I get a genuine certificate, I will file a suit against you.' This is the state of affairs with a famous, senior doctor!

Another example, from Mumbai this time, of an MD in pathology. Acting on the suggestion of the doctor who had referred a patient to him, this pathologist gave a fake report declaring that the patient was diabetic when his blood sugar was normal! A fake pathology report, being given by a MD in pathology!

Why did the concerned general practitioner do this? Because the patient would now become the lifelong patient of the general practitioner. This is what goes on nowadays. And tell me . . . there are private medical colleges which charge lakhs of rupees as capitation fees for admission. Most of those who take admission in such colleges are rolling in money. After graduating from such a college, what does such a doctor think about? He will extract lakhs of rupees from the patients' pockets. This situation must change! It is no longer possible for a poor student to get a medical education. If a poor student is admitted, one can at least hope that he will have some sensitivity towards other human beings. Even this is merely hope, of course, not a certainty. Nowadays one cannot trust anybody.

Just see how we are treating our own professional organizations. The Medical Council of India (MCI), for example. It is widely believed that elections to the MCI are akin to political elections, and only he who has money can get there.

Only those who want to engage in politicking . . . want to inflate their own sense of importance . . . only such people enter these professional organizations, and power is their only motive. There are a few decent people, but they are ineffective. There is no service-orientation left. Only rights are demanded by such associations . . .

right after right. But what about your responsibilities? They have no concern about that, not a jot.

The result is that we were collectively not able to regulate our profession. It was within our ability to impose collective self-regulation, which would have prevented the regulation of doctors being taken over by the government. But that situation no longer remains. That is why we now have no choice but to accept a law like the Clinical Establishments Act and hand over authority to the government. Because it is essential to put an end to the anarchy that currently prevails.

How does anyone claim that we cannot implement 'standard treatment protocols'? Modern medicine is not personalized medicine, as it used to be in ancient times. It has grown into an evidence-based science. With evidence, some standard treatment protocols are now in place. For example, a doctor does not advise test for typhoid on day one of the fever; she waits for the fifth day. There are protocols for treatment of diabetes as well. And in some special cases, you can keep aside the protocol and prescribe another appropriate medicine if required. Nobody is going to penalize you, if you have a convincing rationale for the course you have followed. It is simple to bring in standard treatment protocols. It is certainly possible, and it must happen. Along with this law, those private medical colleges (which charge huge donations) also need to be closed down.

The cost of medicines must come down. That too is possible. It must be mandatory for doctors to prescribe only generic medicines. The third important step is to provide consulting places at low cost. Fees too should be pre-determined. A rate structure could be created. It is certainly possible and it must happen. Because unless we do all of these, no law will have the desired impact.

But what if doctors don't improve even after all this? What can the government do? It can't do anything. Finally, to deal with patients' complaints, there is no alternative but to identify good doctors and create a panel with such doctors. If our professional organizations set up such mechanisms then it would amount to self-regulation by doctors, a direly felt need today.

This is very difficult. Even if a doctor has been grossly negligent ... other doctors cover up for him as a fellow professional. One will have to set up a panel of doctors who will take an objective stand. Bring in any system ... any law ... there is no alternative to setting up such panels, to genuine self-regulation. That is the root of the problem.

All this must be done. Of course, it is a difficult task. But we should start taking steps towards this goal. My sincere best wishes to all of you who are attempting this!

Summing up ...

It is not surprising if you feel bewildered after reading this. This interview, emerging as it does from deep values and feelings, presents before us a noble person like Arjuna who is resisting powerful evil forces. Further, this interview makes us uneasy, since we are likely to think about the past: once upon a time there were such doctors, who cared for patients and knew them personally; this used to be such a service-oriented occupation. The regret that Dr Ajgaonkar feels in his old age makes one uncomfortable. It also evokes an honest anger. 'It should not be so ...' This interview provokes us to question and change this unacceptable state of affairs.

Dr Ajgaonkar is not alone in speaking up about this situation. Another seventy-eight doctors, from various backgrounds, are sharing their experiences and concerns with the reader of these pages. Of all ages, from thirty to eighty, from various parts of the country, from small towns to metros, they want to tell us something that is both revealing and disturbing. They are deeply uneasy as they see the dark shadows multiplying rapidly.

The greatest rot is to be found in hospital transactions. Distortions of the 'noble profession' that are beyond our imagination are being perpetuated. Let us look at some more eye-opening experiences, saying to ourselves, 'Let us know the truth, however disturbing it may be.'

Chapter 2

Malpractices in Private Hospitals

From Dr Ajgaonkar's narration, we have seen how the unimaginable becomes possible, when conscience stops working, and brilliant brains start working in the wrong direction. This is no surprise. A doctor had alerted us to this danger over a century ago. The creator of the world-famous Sherlock Holmes, and himself a physician, stated:

> When a doctor does go wrong he is the first of criminals. He has the nerve and he has the knowledge.
> —Sir Arthur Conan Doyle, *The Speckled Band*

This is unfortunately true. Actually, a doctor's knowledge may be able to save a person's life; it can alleviate a patient's pain. It can ensure that a newborn baby's first cry goes out into the world after a safe delivery. But one essential requirement of a doctor's profession is that the doctor should remain equanimous when treating patients. He has to be careful not to get emotionally involved with any patient; in other words, the doctor must display a calm professionalism. But unfortunately such 'clinical detachment' is sometimes channelized in the service of gross and unscrupulous profiteering.

Some courageous doctors have become whistle-blowers to expose malpractices that occur while patients are admitted in hospitals.

What is the truth about all these malpractices? Some doctors will themselves reveal this 'inside information' now. These doctors are whistle-blowers. They are appealing to all of us: 'See, these are the unacceptable malpractices that are taking place behind closed doors; we are witnessing them, but we alone are unable to change this situation. Now society urgently needs to do something about this.'

Patients need expert medical care at every stage of treatment: making a diagnosis, suggesting various alternative courses of treatment, conducting the treatment through investigations and procedures that the patient prefers and can afford, and informing and counselling the patient properly about the risks that may arise during the course of the treatment. There is always an element of asymmetry in the relationship between doctor and patient. It springs from two sources. There is an information asymmetry and there is a power asymmetry. The asymmetry can be minimized through more awareness in patients but can never be bridged completely. However powerful or rich a person may be, as a patient he or she is always vulnerable. That is the reason why the Hippocratic Oath is given to only the medical profession. The doctor is given a responsibility to also think on behalf of the patient. Unfortunately today we have a situation where this human right is in jeopardy, and we increasingly have to purchase health services like any other commodity. Even in this situation we should have rights as consumers. For instance, appropriate fees should be charged for medical services, and the patient should feel confident that the costs and quality of service are appropriate. But to what extent does this actually happen? To what extent does the private medical sector acknowledge our rights? Our discussions with private doctors revealed the following points.

1. MALPRACTICES DURING DIAGNOSIS

A general practitioner (GP) from a small town observed, 'People have become educated, but there is a loss in that too. Nowadays they have heard of the phrase "Platelet Count" because of the dengue epidemic.

The platelet count drops with any viral fever. I identify such patients in the OPD, and call them daily for a platelet count. Very few need to be admitted, maybe one in a thousand. But many other general practitioners tell educated patients, "See, the count is just 1,50,000 rather than 2 lakh." They give the patient a saline drip, admit him. If the patient is well-off, then straight to the ICU, and a completely avoidable bill of Rs 25,000–30,000 follows!

'There is another peculiar practice. Some level of jaundice among newborns is physiological and normal. Very few babies have to be given treatment with ultraviolet light. But the pathologists give a report: Total bilirubin, 10 mg. They present this report on a printed form that is meant for adult patients. The range shown on that chart indicates the patient has jaundice if the bilirubin level is more than 1 mg. This range is for adults who get jaundice from drinking contaminated water. Almost every newborn has some mild jaundice, and it is dangerous only when the bilirubin level is over 14–16 mg—not 1 mg as in the case of adults.

'Even educated patients are not equipped with the information regarding two different sets of values for the range of bilirubin: one set for adults and one entirely different set for neonates. Instead of using the format meant for neonates, doctors show educated patients the result of a newborn with reference to the adult range and not to the neonatal range. On the adult chart, 1 mg indicates danger, but the actual count is 10 mg! In the neonatal range, 10 mg of bilirubin is normal, while with reference to adult range it looks ten times higher!

'Naturally the parents are frightened and agree to have their normal newborn admitted to the emergency ward, and willingly pay the high costs of the treatment. And over and above that, for the rest of his life the patient sings praises of the doctor, as to how he saved the baby!'

Dr Sanjib Mukhopadhyay, gynaecologist, Kolkata, commented, 'Unethical practices begin right from the stage of writing prescriptions. Listing the qualifications of these doctors, these prescriptions mention degrees that are not recognized by the Medical Council of India or degrees that one [can] get just by paying money. This must stop. This amounts to cheating an ignorant patient!'

2. UNNECESSARY INVESTIGATIONS

Dr Jana, from Shahid Hospital, Chhattisgarh, explained how unscrupulous doctors cheated patients by advising unnecessary tests. 'First they show that the patient has contracted malaria. They show that by a lab test, and give treatment, but the patient does not get better. Then they do another test and show that the patient has typhoid. Doctors are given whatever reports they want by some labs, on payment of a commission.

'The investigations that are made are also often unnecessary. They are not indicated in the textbooks, but they have been euphemistically termed "routine investigations" just to increase the number of investigations required.'

Endorsing this view, Dr Arjun Rajagopalan, a surgeon from Chennai, said, 'It is a rare patient who gets away with just one or two investigations. All the patients I see hold a list of unnecessary tests.'

A pathologist from a metropolitan city revealed how many unnecessary investigations are advised. 'Take typhoid, for example. If the blood test is performed before the fifth day, it does not reveal anything. But it is carried out every alternate day from the first day onwards. The more expensive a test, the more it is prescribed. A sputum examination is generally sufficient to diagnose tuberculosis in the lungs. But the simple reality is that no test can detect it when the tuberculosis is elsewhere in the body—in the stomach, bones, or lymph nodes. But expensive tests like TB Gold and TB Platinum are prescribed. The more expensive the test, the more the commission.'

The pathologist explained the phenomena of 'sink tests': 'This means the sample is just thrown into the sink without testing. The doctor prescribes tests, which by mutual understanding are not actually carried out by the pathologist, who collects the money for the test, and without testing he merely gives a "normal" report. Just one more way of increasing the commission. Many doctors have inadequate knowledge of new tests that are developed—and no desire to learn about them. A new test for TB has been developed. It is clearly written in the test information that it cannot be performed on blood, but only on abdominal and lung fluids. Nevertheless, certain doctors give instructions to perform this test on blood samples. As pathologists, we don't try to enlighten the doctors on such issues, because then their pride is hurt, and then they stop sending us samples.'

A gynaecologist based in a metropolitan city added, 'For pregnant women who are in good health, they incessantly keep prescribing heamograms, kidney function tests and liver function tests.'

Dr Pratibha Kulkarni, a gynaecologist from Pune, gave an instance of when a twenty-two-year-old woman came to her for infertility treatment. 'All investigations were already done. Actually all that was needed was to carry out some basic investigations to verify that there was no big problem. One has to explain to the woman that she should just wait for six to eight months. But all investigations are carried out anyway.

'One woman had an abortion in a big hospital in the month of December because she did not want a child just yet. And then she came to me in April complaining that she could not become pregnant and asking for treatment despite the fact that in the previous month, March, all investigations for infertility had been performed in a big hospital, and she had successfully become pregnant as recently as three months ago. What investigations and treatments could be more unscientific?'

3. Unnecessary Procedures/Operations/Surgeries

A GP from a metropolitan city says, 'After admitting a case of diarrhoea, on the first day itself some doctors administer ten to twelve different kinds of tablets to the patient. I use at most three medicines, which are usually sufficient. But nowadays even when there is no need, lots of medicines are prescribed. When one takes gifts from pharmaceutical companies, the strain is on the patients' pockets, and they end up consuming unnecessary medicines. This is also dangerous!'

Such views are echoed by Dr Shyam Kagal, a physician from Pune. He says, 'I know a gastroenterologist who performs numerous endoscopies on the same patient, when one is sufficient!

He adds, 'The Random Sugar Test is not the ideal test on the basis of which the patients' medication dose can be adjusted. Nevertheless, many physicians perform it.'

This is true of psychiatry as well. Dr Sumit Das, a psychiatrist from Kolkata, reveals, 'In over 80 per cent of cases of depression, when the patient experiences headaches, even though the physician knows that the patient suffers from depression, MRIs and CT scans are performed on all such patients.'

A GP from a big city regrets that 'nowadays even malpractice has become creative. Ingenious schemes are devised for "cut"-based practice. One patient turned up at a hospital and it was decided to perform a hernia operation, as he had been diagnosed with hernia. But it wasn't a hernia at all! Sometimes even when there is no serious ailment, a pretence of surgery is performed. Nothing is really wrong with the patient. But he is given anaesthesia and some stitches are put on the skin, to show that an "operation" has been done. A huge, completely unnecessary bill is charged.'

'Unfortunately, we doctors have pharmaceutical companies as teachers,' laments Dr Gautam Mistry, a cardiologist in Kolkata. 'There is a need to quickly set up an independent mechanism which will play this role, whereby every year doctors can prescribe those medicines only after studying through this system (the system could also be online), not after having been tutored by medical representatives.

'Pharmaceutical companies brazenly promote new medicines to earn profits. Now, attracted by the inducements offered by pharmaceutical companies, even doctors from rural areas are prescribing a new blood-pressure medication which is very expensive. In fact, it is many times more expensive than the effective medicines used earlier. Patients have to take blood-pressure medication for their entire lives, and despite all this, there is not a single piece of evidence demonstrating the efficacy of this medicine! It has become a common practice to bring expensive new medicines to market in place of useful cheaper medicines just to increase profits.

'There is no scientific evidence that these medicines are more effective than the earlier ones. Yet these medicines are promoted,' Dr Mistry adds.

And a city-based gynaecologist explains, 'Many gynaecologists don't want to tediously spend fourteen to sixteen hours taking care of a patient in labour; what is the return [they] would get after devoting so much time? It is more convenient, more profitable—even if not as per the book—for [them] to just perform a quick caesarean and be done with it! This is what is going on.'

Surgery can also be a pitfall for unwary patients. A GP from a metropolitan city observed, 'I know of a case in which, after making a diagnosis of slipped disc (an ailment of the spinal column), no actual surgery was performed and a superficial incision was made, and full operation charges were levied.

'The practice of "cuts" causes another kind of problem. In the past twenty years, I have agreed with and appreciated the technical competence of particular specialists. So much so, that I would take my own mother to them for treatment! Then I should recommend only this specialist's name to my patients, isn't it? But this becomes a problem nowadays. My older patients, who have known me for years, trustingly go to the specialist without asking any questions. But I can see different reactions on the faces of some other patients, when I give such advice . . . Is this general practitioner who is pressing me to go to a particular specialist, taking a cut? I can now spot such a feeling. But I tell such patients immediately . . . it is not necessary for you to go to that particular specialist. Visit anybody you want. But there is always a fear that if this patient mistakenly goes to a totally commercial doctor, and this person recommends all kinds of things, how can I help the patient?'

Nor are these practices confined to big cities. A GP from a small town said, 'Operations for appendicitis/perforations are nowadays casually performed, sometimes even when there is no such condition.

One common unnecessary operation is hysterectomy, which is performed after the patient has been frightened with talk of cancer. All this is increasingly common nowadays. Patients are sent from government hospitals to private hospitals. They are encouraged to shift to the commercial hospital. To ensure this, the private hospital becomes "attached" to the government hospital. Do you understand? Illicit arrangement is made whereby patients from public hospitals are siphoned off by the private hospitals and private practitioners under some pretext or other.'

Pregnant women are particularly susceptible to going in for extra procedures if their doctors advise them to do so. 'Nowadays young doctors, and even some senior ones, quite casually put stitches in the womb of a pregnant woman. Even when it is the first pregnancy,' a gynaecologist practising in a big city revealed. 'The patient just has to complain once of stomach pain, and they perform a sonography, and "manage" the length of the cervix to show that it is short, even when it is normal. With these "managed" sonography reports, doctors scare the patients and tell them—get admitted immediately! Get stitches, or you will have a miscarriage! It's an emergency!

'As for the patients . . . they don't understand and get frightened. And the doctor manages to earn Rs 10,000–15,000. Once stitches have been put in, then that patient usually ends up having a caesarean at the time of delivery. Another extra source of profit.

'Acquiring money is of course a motive. But I also think that most such doctors don't have the required clinical experience, since they have studied in private medical colleges. This can happen. A pregnant woman's stomach could give her pain due to gas . . . but they don't know enough to tell the patient that if one does deep breathing and manages the diet, there will be an improvement. Since they themselves have no experience, they get scared and put in stitches. And since they make money out of this, this becomes the primary method of managing such cases,' they added.

Another lucrative area is paediatrics. 'Vaccinations are so expensive that one doesn't know, for whom one should recommend them,' a paediatrician from a metropolitan city explained. 'If we recommend them, the patients definitely take them. But it places a big burden on their budgets. And if I don't recommend vaccinations, they will certainly ask me, "Who are you to take decisions on our behalf?" All vaccines should be manufactured and supplied by the government. There should be no involvement of private companies.'

As Dr Arjun Rajagopalan, the surgeon from Chennai, pointed out, 'Even in the case of some ordinary business or trade, there is a clear distinction between business conducted ethically and business conducted unethically. Even that sense no longer exists in the medical profession. The practice of cuts/commissions is now routine. As the patients do not have the necessary knowledge, it is the duty of the doctor to look out for the patients' best interests. Taking a cut/commission that is even more than the fee charged for the consultation is totally wrong. But I feel sad when I see that there is no transparency whatsoever left in the private medical sector.

'Every week I come across two to three elderly persons who only need proper spectacles,' said an ophthalmologist working in one of the country's metropolises. 'But they have been told to get operated for cataract (which they don't even have), and they are told the charge is Rs 30,000–40,000. Those who have insurance fall into the trap and go in for the surgery. Those who don't have insurance come to me for a second opinion, and they are saved!

'Every month I get at least two to three cases where the patient has all the paperwork ready. They have been told by some other ophthalmologist to have a cataract surgery, and they have come to me with the required money because someone has recommended me. I examine them and tell them that they have no cataract! This confuses them. They don't know whom to trust. They even harbour the suspicion that I don't understand the issue properly, or that I am scared to perform surgeries. They pressurize me to perform a surgery. But I refuse.'

Patients from the economically weaker sections are specially prone to exploitation, as public health expert, Dr Rajib Dasgupta of Jawaharlal Nehru University, observes, 'Under the Rashtriya

Swasthya Bima Yojana (RSBY, a scheme under which the government purchases the services of private hospitals for poor patients), private doctors diagnose a complicated hernia even when it is a simple hernia, since this fetches them a higher claim. Caesareans help them to earn more money than normal deliveries. And they claim they are forced to do this, because the fees that the government pays are very low! In the case of some surgical procedures, what these doctors claim is true. But missionary hospitals and some other service-oriented hospitals happily implement this scheme. The scheme is a support for them; which also means that the fees are adequate and costs involved to hospitals are affordable.'

4. COMMISSIONS/CUT PRACTICE

A pathologist in a big city shared, 'I did a job in a private set-up for fourteen years. Since the past eight months, I am running my own private practice, having left my lab in the city. A lot of very problematic things are going on nowadays. If I practise ethically, no patients are sent to me. One is expected to do all kinds of things: giving cuts, throwing parties with liquor thrown in, giving doctors whatever reports they want—for example, presenting the Widal Test for typhoid in a way that the doctor can admit the patient, even when he does not have typhoid. Out of 150 doctors whom I am in contact with, there are at the most three or four doctors who find my reports excellent and therefore send me patients without expecting anything in return. Just three or four! Today I am able to manage only because I have other sources of livelihood.'

'Nowadays doctors don't record the [patient's] history properly,' said Dr Punyabrata Goon, a GP in Kolkata. 'They don't even examine the patient. They just write out a list of investigations. Because they get a commission for doing that. Almost all the laboratories in our area give 50 per cent commission and almost all the doctors accept these commissions. For many doctors, the money earned through commissions is much more than that earned from fees. In our area, the commission rates are: X-rays 25 per cent, and 33 per cent for MRIs and CT scans.'

A paediatrician in Delhi, Sanjay Bhatnagar explained how the system is harmful: 'I don't take cuts. I tell patients to go wherever they please to get the investigations done. The patient then goes to his own GP and asks him where he should do the test. The general practitioner gives him a slip referring him to a pathologist, and gets a cut for this. But I have no faith in that report. Unfortunately I cannot even tell the patient where the problem lies.'

A big city physician explains how even those who refuse to take cuts are drawn into the system: 'The routine hospital charges actually include the cuts. And even though I do not take cuts, this extra amount is not reduced from my patients' bills. Given this situation, many people ask me what I achieve by not taking cuts. I don't know. I consider taking cuts to be unethical and I don't take them. When I inquired, I was told that the hospital transfers the cuts that I do not take to a separate fund, which is used for emergency expenditures!'

'Nowadays the charges in the medical sector have increased to the extent that even I wonder whether I will be able to afford them in future,' lamented Dr Pratibha Kulkarni, a gynaecologist from Pune.

Most private hospitals, whether big or small, are part of this system, though the latter are more transparent. A GP practising in a metropolis explained, 'The running charges in a small hospital are the same as in a multi-speciality hospital. But in the multi-speciality hospitals to which I send my patients, there is a rate chart, there is transparency. In small hospitals, protocols and rules are not followed for diagnosis and treatment. They charge whatever they want, and they extract as much money as they can from patients. I will not support the practice of cuts. Neither do I take cuts. Some general practitioners say that there is an outrageous disparity between their bills and those charged by specialists and hospitals. People do not pay even a little extra money to a general practitioner. But they will pay whatever specialists and hospitals demand. Then what is wrong with taking a share of that money? But I don't agree with this practice. Why should I cut into my patients' pockets when I refer a case that

I cannot manage, to a specialist or hospital? No. Cuts cannot be justified whatever the reason behind them. Yes, one thing should change: One should ensure that hospitals and specialists levy only reasonable charges—we need a system where the current anarchy does not continue.'

The cuts come under all sorts of heads. Dr Suchitra, a GP from Chennai, revealed, 'I happily refused to become a person who accepts commissions. Once a laboratory PRO visited me. He offered me a certain percentage as "IC". I did not even know what IC stood for. Apparently, it means "Interpretation Charges". What blasted interpretation? There is nothing in the laboratory report on which I can use my knowledge. This was nothing but a cut under a cute name. I refused, and told them to give the cut to the patient.'

'The way the "cuts" system works is, it actually operates against those who refuse to take them,' Dr Hemant Kotwal, a Nasik-based radiologist, said. 'Actually, after 25–30 years of practice, we should install newer technologies and facilities here. But then it does not work out financially for me—if I take a loan for lakhs of rupees to buy a machine, and then do not pay cuts to get the patients. Hence I end up with no choice, except deciding not to buy the machine! From another perspective, this too is unfair to the patients.'

'The very objectives and motivations for joining the medical profession have changed,' said Dr George Mathai, a physician from Alibag, Maharashtra. 'Nowadays the only purpose of joining the medical profession is to make as much money as one can, with as little work as one can get away with. On one hand, cuts are given. Yet, if a patient comes directly without a referring doctor, he is not given any concession.'

As a gynaecologist practising in a big city pointed out, 'There is one more reason why cuts are given. Doctors who take cuts for every patient they refer will criticize and slander a clean doctor, till his reputation is ruined. Thus those who do not give cuts, come under pressure. To avoid this, one has to give cuts! One doctor actually lied to my patient, saying that I take cuts from these doctors! What am I to do when faced with such people? I am helpless. One even sees plenty of doctors who refer their own relatives; they allow for inflation of expenses, and then ask for a cut.'

The pervasiveness of cuts draws in all those linked to hospitals. The above-mentioned gynaecologist adds, 'Ambulance drivers and autorickshaw drivers also get a cut. Nowadays doctors admit patients in their own clinics, even when they know the case is beyond their competence. They keep the patient with them until the condition deteriorates and there is no choice but referring the patient. A huge bill is run up. Once the case has gone out of control, they send the patient to a corporate hospital. They get commissions in that process too.'

Dr Shyam Ashtekar, from Dindori in the Nasik district, suggests the cuts should be passed on to the specialist, not the patient: 'I feel that it may be all right to have a formal system of a 10 or 20 per cent cut, that is uniform and legal. But one thing to ensure is that this amount is deducted from the specialists' share. The patient should not have to pay extra.'

The surgeon continues, 'When setting up a new hospital, the hospital owners assign space to a pathology lab and a pharmacy. They take Rs 50–75 lakh as deposit from these units. So nowadays you don't even need to take a loan from a bank to raise money for setting up a hospital. Naturally, after this deal, no regulation of the pathology lab or the pharmacy is possible. The labs and pharmacies even ensure that the money they (the hospital's owners) have kept as deposit is recovered from the patients' pockets. In order to achieve high returns, of course, no importance is given to issues like whether the procedure is necessary or not, or any ethical considerations. Patients are admitted unnecessarily. Earlier, we used to treat babies with simple packets of ORS (electrolyte powder against dehydration) at the OPD (outdoor patients) level, without admitting them. But now in such hospitals, these babies are admitted. Children who are playing happily are admitted to hospitals! Even the parents insist upon it.

'Now surgery has become very expensive. Instead of just three or four, eight to ten medicines are prescribed. In return, pharmaceutical companies pay regular instalments of Rs 50,000 to 1 lakh to doctors.

Even if you give absolutely rational treatment, some pharmaceutical companies are willing to pay you. That is the extent of the profit margin they have.

'A lipoma (small, non-cancerous, fatty growth) operation was quoted to cost Rs 50,000. Then it was said that with new technology, and shorter duration of operation, it would be performed for Rs 1,10,000. Finally the price came down to the actual cost of Rs 20,000! This means there is no rate of standardization. If I need surgery, I hope the public hospital has the necessary facilities. I would rather go there than pay these inflated charges!

'In an emergency, nothing is done as per rational guidelines. The whole situation is troublesome for the hospital that does not take a cut for referrals. If we have referred a patient, people assume that we have received a cut for our referral. So people come to us asking for a share from that cut they assume we have received from the bill of that seriously ill patient!

'Apart from the cut, smaller hospitals are going to face one other crunch. They are unable to get qualified doctors. These hospitals will not survive much longer, certainly not in rural areas. One cannot not get an MBBS degree holder as duty doctor for a hospital. One gets plenty of BAMS (Bachelor in Ayurvedic Medicine) degree holders and one can train them. But there is no legal protection if you do this. What are we to do?'

The surgeon also mentions, 'There is a government scheme for the poor—the Rashtriya Swasthya Bima Yojana. The rates set under this plan are too low, and doctors cannot afford to do procedures under this scheme.'

According to Dr Rajendra Malose, a GP from Chandwad in the Nasik district, 'Nowadays one gets Rs 30,000–40,000 just for referring a patient for angioplasty. Dead patients continue to be kept on ventilators, until the anger of their relatives cools off. As soon as an accident takes place on the highway, seven or eight of these fellows go running to the site. "This one is mine, this one is mine," they say as they lift the patients. Is it a good thing that they promptly take such patients to orthopaedic wards of corporate hospitals? Or a bad thing?

'And then in doctors' parties there are colourful discussions about how a certain "lamb" was caught . . . and slaughtered. "It's the slack season now" kind of stuff. They are saddened when people in society around them are in good health.'

However, some doctors insist that despite the pervasive lack of scruples, it is still possible to practise honestly. A GP from one of India's metropolises says, 'If you are ethical, once people are convinced about your ethical behaviour—then a GP's practice can be successful without giving any cuts. I practise in an educated environment; I am in touch only with ethical doctors. They are attached to certain hospitals. In the past twenty years, I have not met a single bad specialist . . . '

Though, as Pune physician Dr H.V. Sardesai observes, 'I did not get a cheque for my cut like Dr Bawaskar did. I am sure that you must have heard his case from newspapers. Dr Bawaskar, a famous physician from Mahad, got the cut by cheque! But I know for certain that this kind of cut practice is going on.'

'Many doctors have clearly decided that there is no choice but to practise medicine as if one is running a business,' says Dr Vinay Kulkarni, an HIV and skin specialist from Pune. 'They are involved in cut practice right from the beginning. After the advent of large and corporate hospitals, these practices have increased further. Malpractices are committed in a number of ways. For one, certain procedures are carried out even when knowledge and skill for them is lacking. The patient loses due to this. For another, both your and my share is extracted from the patient's pocket. And a third way is to say, "This procedure has been done" when it's not been done at all, and to take money for what has never been done.'

Patients are exploited at every turn. Dr Subhash Patil, a gynaecologist from Sangli, Maharashtra, describes how even going to a hospital of their choice can be a problem: 'At 2 a.m., autorickshaw drivers here tell patients directly, "I don't know the hospital you are talking about." Because he will take the patient only to the hospital that offers him a cut. Now even autorickshaw drivers are on the lists of those receiving cuts from doctors.

'It's the destiny of every patient, which determines whether he will be in the hands of an honest doctor (there are very few of those anyway) or in the hands of a businessman. After all, how is a patient to know which doctor is honest? There is no means by which an ordinary person can find out!'

5. LACK OF REGULATION: QUESTIONABLE DEGREES AND TREATMENT WITHOUT REQUIRED KNOWLEDGE

'They do not teach laser treatment in our medical colleges,' explained a skin specialist practising in a big city. 'We learn by trial and error, experimenting on patients. These machines are forced upon us by other countries. They have been tested on foreigners. There is no study on people of Indian ethnicity and skin colour. Mistakes happen, and once one has got a laser machine, there is a rush to recover the cost. Even when there is no need, when it has no treatment value, patients are fed to the machine.'

Qualifications are often misrepresented. An ophthalmologist in a medium-sized city says, 'In one small town, an "ophthalmologist" with a questionable qualification for eye surgery performs cataract operations. There is no regulation. Who is allowed to operate? Optometrists test people's eyes, and also treat people. They collect and channelize patients to corporate hospitals.'

'I feel that some of these people with BHMS and BAMS degrees (homeopathic and Ayurvedic medicine degrees respectively) have become a nuisance,' said an ophthalmologist based in a big city. 'They just copy my prescriptions word for word. I am an MS (Master of Surgery). I make a diagnosis after numerous examinations and only then do I prescribe medicine.

'I had a patient, a four-year-old girl. Since the past one year, her eyes would become red from time to time. The mother was taking her to a BHMS doctor. That fellow was repeatedly prescribing steroid drops, and the mother was administering them. For a full year, the same drops, given many times over (steroid eye drops should not be given for long periods since they can cause cataract).

'Later she came to me saying that her daughter now cannot see properly. She had developed cataract. I performed a cataract surgery on a four-year-old girl!

'This is the kind of things that some BHMS doctors can be up to.'

Doctors who try to work professionally have an uphill task. A public health specialist from one of the metropolises says, 'I will tell you a real story of my batch mate. He was the topper in our batch, very sharp. He did his MD in paediatrics from a renowned college in the city and set up his private clinic. When he saw other private paediatricians prescribing Lomotil (medicine for diarrhoea with potential serious side effects) to small children, for whom it is clearly prohibited, he decided that he would not get into this kind of a rat race. Our patients have a herd mentality and follow the crowd. They don't look at the doctor's qualifications. That is why new doctors often try to employ all possible means to draw patients, showing quick results. Otherwise the doctor may have no patients, and may have to go hungry.

'This bright doctor's practice, though rational, was not doing well, and he finally shut it down ... rather than engage in criminal practices just to attract crowds of patients, he emigrated to Canada.'

6. Inflated Bills

A big city dentist poses this question: 'How can we ourselves determine the value of our knowledge? Can I decide my profit margin as I feel like? If medical service is really a service, then how is it that the prices set by the doctors themselves become unaffordable to most people?

'Although taking an X-ray of a single tooth would suffice, X-rays of ten teeth are taken just to inflate the bill from Rs 50 to Rs 500.'

'Nowadays the patient is not the central point of medical practice,' says Dr Sanjay Nagral, a Mumbai surgeon. 'First, one thinks of one's own benefit. While one pursues this, in passing there may be some benefit to the patient. The criteria by which society measures a doctor's success has also changed, as has the criteria by which doctors judge themselves. Now the successful doctor is one who has a big car, and earns a lot of money! Due to this, everything is now dictated by the logic of the market. The very structure of private medical practice has now become such that there is no place left for ethics.

'As a soldier pushed into war, in order to save his life, advances firing heavily and indiscriminately, so too a doctor entering the private medical sector now starts his practice with a business-minded and market-oriented perspective. Obviously, any solutions that are to emerge must be such that reform the system.'

The costs of treatment are unregulated. A big city-based physician said, 'One does not know exactly what one should define as inflated charges. The largest amounts are charged for surgery and procedures. This was the case twenty years ago as well. I took a patient to a cancer specialist in Mumbai. He didn't even examine the patient properly and wrote out a prescription for medicines that were outdated. They were not available even in the pharmacy below his own clinic! He changed the medicines after I went back to him. And he charged Rs 6000 as consulting fee!

'I sent a patient to a surgeon to get a small incision done, a ten-minute procedure using ether spray. He came back and said, "They are demanding Rs 40,000." What is the basis of such exorbitant charges? Who knows what is the rationale behind these charges? Each doctor decides the price himself. Who is there to decide that certain charges are unrealistic and inflated?

'Nowadays we have one hospital charging Rs 30,000 for a specific surgery, and another one charging Rs 60,000 for the same surgery. Why? Just like that . . . '

A skin specialist based in a big city adds, 'They quote Rs 25,000 for chemotherapy and then later present a bill for Rs 65,000. There are many such examples. Actually, this is a completely planned treatment with no variation. There is no scope to raise the prices.

Why would one take advantage of the helplessness of a cancer patient in this manner?'

'The proportion of caesarean deliveries in our private hospitals is very high,' says Dr Shirish Patwardhan, a gynaecologist from Pune and former vice president, FOGSI (Organization of Obstetricians and Gynaecologists). 'In Pune city, it is around 50 per cent and in the Pimpri–Chinchwad area it is 25 per cent. I feel that all private gynaecologists should put up a board stating the percentage of caesarean deliveries in his hospital. Then, if a woman wants a caesarean, she can go to the hospital which has the highest percentage. And if a woman prefers a normal delivery, she can go to the hospital which has a low percentage of caesarean deliveries.'

'Some doctors actually commit theft in hospitals,' a big-city surgeon reveals. 'Should a surgeon steal a saline bottle? Of course not. But he does. The patient is helpless. You will charge whatever you want, because you are famous. This is just not right.'

'Infertility treatments are particularly lucrative,' a gynaecologist from a big city explained. 'In big cities now, infertility treatment has become an even easier route to earn money than hysterectomies were earlier. It is known that in such procedures, the success rate is low. So it is a safe game. Even if there is no success, nobody blames you. But to whom should one recommend IVF? When should one recommend it? No proper guidance is given. One does not even consider whether the patient can afford it.'

Dr Chandrakant Pandav, professor and head at the Centre for Community Medicine, AIIMS, New Delhi reflected, 'Nowadays private practice is something done only to earn money, not to provide service; making more and more money, to pay the instalments on your Mercedes and for your foreign trips. That is the only purpose of private practice nowadays. Now we have moved from the Science of Health to the Science of Exploitation.'

According to Dr Satish Gosain, a GP in Delhi, 'By and large, an angioplasty should cost around Rs 1,50,000. But I have seen hospitals charging Rs 3–3.5 lakh.'

7. MAKING MONEY THROUGH PRESCRIBING MEDICINES INAPPROPRIATELY

'Pharmacies that operate within hospitals must be closed immediately. (Such drug stores often charge inflated rates for medicines from patients in the hospital who are a "captive audience"),' said a big city-based skin specialist. 'Now even patients ask me, "Doctor, tell us right now where we can buy your medicine . . . so that I can go straight there." This must be stopped.'

8. MISCELLANEOUS

'Combining private practice with rational, ethical treatment has become an uneconomic proposition,' concluded Dr Vandana Prasad, a Delhi-based paediatrician. 'If you see the prescriptions from private paediatricians, they contain only treatment. No history is written down. Even the diagnosis is not written. As for growth charts, nobody uses them. All this is unforgivable.

'The shocking truth is that some paediatricians even advise mothers not to breastfeed their babies! This is saddening. That is, mothers are ready to breastfeed and doctors tell them not to do so. This is criminal. It is an example of the way doctors want to exert their power over patients. The plan behind giving such advice is to prohibit something the mother can do herself, and to take control. Because now the mother will come every month to ask the doctor how she should feed powder milk to her baby. Besides, there is of course the influence of powder-milk manufacturing companies behind such advice.'

But it is not that corruption is only found in private practice. Government hospitals, too, are not immune, according to a surgeon from a megacity. 'There is a difference between government hospitals and private hospitals. One faces many practical difficulties while working in a government hospital. One does not have the kind of freedom one has in private practice. Hence, one's own progress may get hampered. It is not as if there is always more corruption in government hospitals. But the overall system is conducive to corruption. Therefore, everybody feels that private practice is a more convenient system.'

Dr L.R. Murmu, professor of surgery at AIIMS, Delhi, points out the merciless exploitation of terminal cancer patients in the private health care sector. He illustrates, 'Sometimes we [working in a large public hospital] tell one of our patients that the cancer has spread extensively through his body, hence an operation is not possible. There is no further cure that can be attempted. Then the patient goes to a private facility. There they do some smooth talking, play on the emotions of the family, and perform an operation on a patient when it is certain to fail—and thus make a lot of money.

'Nowadays I tell my patients not to rely only on our opinion. They should certainly get a second opinion from a private practitioner. That is the patient's right. But be smart when you get a second opinion. From my side, I will teach you three specific questions about your case, and the correct answers. Ask the doctor these three questions. Believe what he advises, only if he answers these three questions correctly. My experience is that they mostly avoid answers to such direct questions. All they do is rouse emotions through smooth and evasive talk. In that case, you know that such a doctor does not give appropriate advice!

'Many patients have operations in private hospitals. There, for example, after a colectomy operation (removal of colon), the histopathology of the removed tissue is not performed. To make sure I ask the patient, "After being advised to do it, did you still not do it in order to save money?" And the patient replies that he was not told anything about such a test! This practice of not performing tissue histopathology is rampant in the private sector. It is completely unscientific and reflects negligence.'

Observing the widespread rot in the private health care sector, Dr Mandar Paranjape, a pathologist from Pune, and taking a cue from the particular phase of normal sleep as taught in the medical curriculum, comments wittily, 'The short form of Rational Ethical Medical Practice is REM practice. REM Sleep is a part of our sleep, a part during which we dream. Will REM practice similarly remain only a dream? That is the question that worries me.'

Summing up . . .

This is what is going on in the medical sector today. Such anarchy in a sphere that deals with questions of life and death, such naked pursuit of profit! There is no regulation based on qualifications, nor any regulation regarding how private practice is to be conducted. One can do whatever one wants. This situation has gone out of control. These quotes are honest admissions by doctors, of the frequent malpractices in hospitals. Let us end this chapter with something that one of these doctors said in his interview:

Whenever there is any discussion of the malpractices in the medical profession, doctors' associations reply that every profession has a few black sheep. Maybe some such rare elements are involved in such unethical acts. But overall they claim the medical profession is clean! But I feel that we will now need a microscope to find any white sheep that remain! This is the level to which this profession has sunk.

—Dr George Mathai, physician, Alibag,
Raigarh district, Maharashtra

Chapter 3

The Toxic Influence of Pharmaceutical Companies

The perception that pharmaceutical companies have a vice-like grip over many doctors is widespread today. As soon as they graduate from medical college, medical representatives of pharmaceutical companies take charge of them. The young doctors forget all that they have learnt. They ignore the fact, for instance, that fever can be treated with plain paracetamol. They come to think only in terms of branded products, which cost five times as much, and it is medical representatives who introduce them to these new medicines. Various schemes are offered—ranging from trips to Singapore and America, to, as one ophthalmologist informed us, vests and briefs to lure the doctors into the pharma-firms' sphere of influence.

Pharmaceutical companies often cover the costs of conferences in India and abroad, which promote new medicines and new technologies. Many doctors are willingly 'seduced'. So much so that in one city, the local branch of the doctors' association decided by secret ballot that henceforth all their Continuing Medical Education (CME) workshops would not be conducted through subscription from the members on subjects of their choice. Instead, they would be sponsored by pharmaceutical companies, and the subjects covered are now often chosen by the companies themselves.

Through such methods pharmaceutical companies have managed to purchase a majority of doctors—MBBS doctors, specialists and even super-specialists, as well as homeopathic and Ayurvedic doctors who are not formally trained in allopathic pharmacology. The end result is a frightening situation of market-driven anarchy and chaos!

In a doctor's toolkit to fight disease, the most important tool is medicine. Pharmaceutical companies and doctors should complement each other. Today, one cannot think of a situation where one exists without the other. But it may be worth remembering that just a hundred and fifty years ago, there were no pharmaceutical companies. Doctors had at their disposal just a few self-prepared remedies like opium and mercury. Patients were sometimes anaesthetized by giving a blow on the head. Over the past hundred years, we have made tremendous progress in medical science and technology. But the fact that major commercialization of medical technology has taken place is also an unwanted reality. Pharmaceutical companies began to enter the market with newer drugs, and in no time at all the arithmetic of profit was all that mattered, which overruled all other considerations.

It is the patient who buys medicine; the money comes out of the patient's pocket. But the patient has no control over this purchase. When someone goes to the market to buy soap, they know about the colour, scent and price of the soap they want to buy. The grocer does not decide whether the consumer should buy Lifebuoy or Lux; the consumer asks for it. But when it comes to buying medicines, things are different. This is not like buying soap—the patient can hardly decide which medicine they should buy . . . 'Give me this or that antibiotic.' No, this has always been decided by the patient's doctor in the past, and will continue to be decided by the doctor. This is not a decision which the patient is ever likely to take independently. Therefore, it will always remain the doctor's responsibility to take the patient's best interest into account when prescribing any medicine.

This monopoly that doctors have, in deciding on the purchase of particular medicines, is an important basis for pharmaceutical companies to maximize their profits by often unethical means. All that the companies have to do is to gain control over the doctors by dangling various temptations in front of them.

1. INDUCEMENTS

Dr Satish Gosain, a general practitioner in Delhi, says, 'Doctors have now become servants of the pharmaceutical companies.'

A general surgeon from a big city comments, 'Don't even mention pharmaceutical companies. They have purchased us . . .

'We had organized a conference. We decided that each doctor would pay a subscription towards the expenses. We had thought that we would not take any sponsorship from pharmaceutical companies. But finally we ended up making hotel bookings for only around 100 out of the 1200 doctors who attended. Practically all the other doctors who attended the conference allowed the pharmaceutical companies to pay for their hotel bookings, transport, and food arrangements.

'The doctors must maintain a sense of ethics and probity. But that does not usually happen.'

'As soon as a medical student becomes a doctor, the pharmaceutical companies take control. There is not even any sense of remorse that accepting gifts is a blow to their prestige and ethics. On the contrary, doctors consider these gifts as a right,' says Dr Jana, from Shahid Hospital in Chhattisgarh.

Dr H.V. Sardesai, practising physician in Pune, adds, 'Pharmaceutical companies take doctors on foreign trips. They make all the arrangements. And there just is a pretence of doing some study on these trips. Unfortunately there are many doctors who enjoy all this.

'Why is there such a large difference between prices of the same medicine, charged by different pharmaceutical companies, when the chemical used is the same? There should not be such a vast difference!

'There have been numerous advertisements in which various actresses were depicted using Lux soap. Every young woman would buy this soap. Now pharmaceutical companies disseminate similar advertisements. These advertisements tell fresh, young doctors: "See, eminent doctors prescribe our medicines!" The junior doctors fall prey to these advertisements . . .

'Today even many senior doctors prescribe eight to ten medicines, when a few tablets would suffice. There is no doubt that the pharmaceutical companies have promoted this practice.'

A gynaecologist from Kolkata, Dr Sanjib Mukhopadhyay, shares, 'Now smart medical representatives of pharmaceutical companies "teach" those who are trained as doctors! I tell these doctors, "You are the cream of society; don't you feel ashamed to learn from these medical representatives?" Many organizations and associations of medical professionals are hand in glove with these pharmaceutical companies. The question is: why have we allowed pharmaceutical companies to become our teachers?

'The result of this is that doctors do not treat the disease—they treat the complaint. And the pharmaceutical companies too are selling medicines that alleviate the complaint.

'Look at the names of some of these medicines: Nopotty—for what? Diarrhoea! Isn't this trivialization of medical science?

'Even though this is not recommended in any textbook, many gynaecologists merrily prescribe a medication called Progesterone even for normal pregnancies! Actually, pregnancy is a natural process. But in order to benefit the pharmaceutical companies, we doctors have now converted it into an illness. It is obvious why doctors are so eager to patronize pharmaceutical companies.

'Now we have to look with suspicion even at things which are presented as "backed by evidence". Under the influence of the West and pharmaceutical companies, some products are coming to the forefront, because of the claim that they are evidence-based. What if they tell us that we should use a certain antibiotic which is very expensive, in preference to the established, cheaper antibiotic I currently use, and of which I have had a positive experience? Do I recommend it to the poor rickshaw driver? It will ruin him. I will not use that new antibiotic for the rickshaw driver, even if it is supposedly evidence-based.

'I once asked the members of all-India bodies of medical professionals why they hide the fact that pharmaceutical companies have sponsored them to attend this conference. Each doctor who has come with such sponsorship should wear a tie of that company! Why are they coy about this? At least one will be able to identify those few who have come on their own money! Why is there no such transparency?

'I have come to know that the senior office-bearers of many doctors' associations and organizations in India have been bought up by particular pharmaceutical companies. By not publicly revealing this, they are fooling their own members.'

Dr Rajendra Malose, a general practitioner, from Chandwad, in the Nasik district, comments, 'Some pharmaceutical companies have been advertising "Emergency Contraceptives" for over-the-counter sale. No medical body objected. Even today nobody objects. These tablets are being used by people in an incorrect, half-baked fashion. Pharmaceutical companies have today made puppets of the doctors—literally, puppets that dance to their tune.'

'Pharmaceutical companies routinely promote allopathic medicines to doctors who do not have an MBBS degree. How does this happen?' a super-specialist from a big city wonders. 'I never accept sponsorship by pharmaceutical companies. I spend my own money to attend conferences. Once when I went for a conference, there were no rooms in any of the hotels in the city—they had all been booked by the pharmaceutical companies! What was I to do . . . I was left with no alternative but to stay in a hotel booked by one of the pharmaceutical companies!'

'Some of my doctor friends boast to me that they have travelled the world, sponsored by pharmaceutical companies. One was telling me with pride that even their shirts, pants, vests and underwear are given by pharmaceutical companies!' says an ophthalmologist from a medium-sized city.

Dr Suchitra, a general practitioner in Chennai, mentions, 'The pharmaceutical companies offered to sponsor me for a conference, but I refused. I usually prescribe generic medicines or cheap, branded medicines. But the interesting thing is that once these pharmaceutical companies realized I don't prescribe their medicines, they stopped visiting me.

'I have been practising for thirty years. I have not given any "cuts",' a super-specialist from a metropolis shares. 'I did not encourage pharmaceutical companies. I change the medicines prescribed to my patients, prescribing cheaper medicines if expensive medicines have been prescribed. And what a big difference this makes to the patient! Sometimes the cost is reduced as much as Rs 35–40 per tablet! Patients are often unnecessarily prescribed expensive brands of medicines, for years on end, sometimes for life. The hapless patient keeps taking these medicines.

'Once, four medical representatives visited me with their bosses. They tried to convince me that I should not replace their brands, while prescribing cheaper brands to patients. We discussed the matter for an hour and their argument was that their company does a lot of research, on which they spend crores of rupees. That is why their brand is more expensive by Rs 30 per tablet.

'After they had finished their speech, I took Rs 1000 out of my pocket and handed it to one of the bosses. Surprised, he asked me what this was for. I answered: "You are doing such good work for humankind. This is my small contribution!"

'After that I emphatically told them that I would help them, but how could I do this at the patients' expense without telling the patients? Of course, they had no answer to that.'

A big-city surgeon remarks, 'Pharmaceutical companies sponsor conferences where nobody bothers to listen to the lectures. Doctors just go to the stalls, and collect gifts. They enjoy the free drinks. It is a filthy business. What can one say?'

'Medical representatives influence the doctors. One of them offered me a trip to Singapore. I refused and told him that I would go at my own expense, and when I wanted,' said a general practitioner from a big city.

A super-specialist from a metropolitan city also shares, 'The medical representatives are really persistent; they don't leave you alone. Earlier, I would get angry at them. One of them pleaded with me, "Sir, you are the only one left. The other doctors, like you, who would earlier not take gifts, have all gradually succumbed. That's why I am now meeting you too." Since then, I don't get angry with them.

'Recently, a medical representative brought along a diamond necklace as a gift, worth Rs 1 lakh.

'I asked him, "What's this?"

'"A diamond necklace, sir."

'"For whom?"

'"It's for your wife."

'Controlling my temper, I asked him, "How do you dare to put a necklace on my wife's neck?"

'The poor fellow was taken aback. "It is you ... you will put the necklace on your wife's neck."

'Giving it back to him, I told him in a calm voice, "If that is so, then I will buy it with my own money. That is, if she wants a necklace at all!"

'The poor fellow left with the necklace.'

Dr Sumit Das, a psychiatrist from Kolkata notes, 'Pharmaceutical companies exist to do business and make profits. But what about doctors? They too put pressure on pharmaceutical companies, telling them, "If I prescribe your medicines, send me on a tour to Europe."

'In the field of psychiatry, pharmaceutical companies bring out new medications every day. There is no evidence that the new medications are better than the cheaper and effective medications that are already in use. And keep in mind the fact that our patients don't take these medications for just a few days, but often for months or even longer. Yet these unnecessarily expensive medicines are sold and also prescribed.'

'Pharmaceutical companies could have donated money to our department and our institution by cheque. But instead of doing that, I would repeatedly be offered personal gifts, foreign trips, etc. Those salesmen would tell me openly that they are willing to spend on an individual, not on the institution,' comments a general surgeon from a metropolitan city.

A paediatrician from a metropolitan city suggests, 'The practice of pharma companies sponsoring doctors for conferences and CME (Continuing Medical Education) workshops must be stopped immediately.'

A gynaecologist from a big city observes, 'The area manager of a pharmaceutical company once paid me a visit along with his army of representatives. He asked me why I regularly use a certain product manufactured by them.

'I answered, "It is cheap, it is effective. That's why."

'He was confused. He asked me in bewilderment, "Madam, we never give you any gifts."

'I replied, "There is no need for that."

'He just could not believe it. He kept asking, "How can this be, madam? Please tell me the reason."

'This is the ridiculous situation that prevails. This is the reality.'

A paediatrician from a big city mentions, 'Our branch [of a doctors' association] was functioning well. We would organize CME workshops with our own funds. Gradually, the pharmaceutical companies pushed their way in. From 1995 onwards they began to organize their own CME workshops. Earlier, we would focus on the issues of importance that we had decided upon. But then the pharmaceutical companies began to select only those topics that would help them promote their new drugs. The workshops were free, with liquor thrown in. Finally the doctors in our city decided that all workshops henceforth would be organized by the pharmaceutical companies. I would ask them why they couldn't spend Rs 1000 per year on their own education. Why do you want it free? Finally, through a secret ballot, my opposition was set aside and the basic principles of our [doctors' association] branch were changed in favour of the pharma companies. Obviously, I withdrew from it. Now all workshops in our city are conducted by pharmaceutical companies.'

'A rampant malpractice is in the area of prescribing vaccines—it is organized, and takes place on a large-scale in planned fashion. The practitioner gets a cut on the Maximum Retail Price (MRP). The more expensive the vaccine, the higher the cut. The cut is even more than the consultation fee. The doctor gets both—the cut from the company and the fee from the patient,' notes Dr Vandana Prasad, a paediatrician from Delhi.

'The pharmaceutical companies are like a pack of wolves. They keep pestering you and encourage you to accept some incentives. Once you take anything from them, they immediately become arrogant. Now they begin to ask you directly, "Why don't you prescribe our medicine?" They start dictating terms, and because you have accepted money and gifts, you are morally bound to them,' Dr Sanjay Bhatnagar, a paediatrician from Delhi, also shares.

A surgeon from a megacity mentions, 'The government cannot provide funds, and if the pharmaceutical companies therefore sponsor conferences in a transparent manner, there is nothing wrong with it. The MCI wanted to do something about this.'

2. Aggressive, Predatory Marketing

A skin specialist from a big city says, 'The pharmaceutical companies have created mayhem. Things like conference sponsorship by drug companies must be stopped. The MCI is aware of the problem, but there are lots of loopholes that can be exploited. Nowadays, doctors take money from pharmaceutical companies and prescribe ten to twenty medicines in a single prescription. There is always an antioxidant tablet prescribed, whether it serves any purpose or not.'

A skin specialist from Kolkata, Dr Jayant Das also remarks, 'Now pharmaceutical companies are resorting to a new strategy.

'For example, they don't even produce Doxycycline (an established antibiotic) capsules, which cost less than Re 1 per capsule. Instead, they add a useless component like lactobacillus with Doxycycline, and then sell each of those capsules for Rs 5. And when the ordinary, cheap Doxycycline capsule is not even available in the market by design, one has no choice but to prescribe the expensive medicine. This is happening without any check with respect to many medications. One company recently withdrew a medication available for Rs 2. They made some token changes in the formulation and the same tablet is now sold by them for Rs 15!'

Another skin specialist from a big city observes, 'Pharmaceutical companies try to give money to doctors under the pretext of conducting studies on their medicines. Such bogus clinical trials are conducted openly. The doctors lure the patients with the promise that the stated medication has come from abroad, and if you want to have it free, you would have to just sign this form, that's all! Please sign here. Doctors collect the signatures on the forms. Sometimes they just fill up the details. Once they have given the papers for ten to twelve cases (even without prescribing the medication) they get a cheque from the pharmaceutical company.

'If one puts an end to the money pharmaceutical companies spend on doctors, medicines will definitely become much cheaper. That must be ensured, for the benefit of patients. Doctors should be legally compelled to prescribe only generic medicines.'

A general surgeon from a big city offers, 'Take the example of Lactulose, which is used to treat constipation. It costs about Rs 180 for 200 ml, that is, around Rs 900 a litre. This is a by-product of the sugar industry. Actually, this should cost less than sugar, i.e., less than Rs 60 per kg. Elderly people will be taking this for years together. Shouldn't the prices of such medicines be regulated? No. The loot continues.'

'In almost 60 per cent of the cases, I discontinue the medicines mentioned in prescriptions given by other doctors, because they are not needed. There are very few MBBS doctors in my block. Most of the general practitioners are BHMS (homeopaths) and BAMS (Ayurvedic). They are not involved in the scientific rationale of allopathic medicines. They often don't even go into the details of diagnosis. They just prescribe the medicines as the pharma companies have taught them; without much thought, whatever they feel like,' says Dr Rajiv Dhamankar, a paediatrician from Alibag, Maharashtra.

A gynaecologist from a big city also remarks, 'Pharmaceutical companies create artificial "waves". Which scientific report is one to accept as true? Nowadays, there is a wave of prescribing vitamin D. The consumption has increased exponentially worldwide. But there are also some reports which claim that vitamin D can lead to cancer. This vitamin is not expelled through the urine like other vitamins, but accumulates in the body. It has side effects. What is true? This report of increased cancer due to vitamin D, or the marketing by pharmaceutical companies?'

A practising surgeon in a megacity comments, 'The unscientific treatments that one sees are largely related to the over-prescription of antibiotics. But where are the protocols to curb this malpractice?'

As a big-city ophthalmologist explains, 'A new antibiotic is introduced with a very specific use. But the pharmaceutical company has a target. Ninety per cent of this target is met through non-allopathic doctors who are not trained in modern pharmacology, who are convinced to prescribe the new antibiotic by any means. They casually write advanced antibiotics even for a simple cold. The result? Simply that widespread resistance to the advanced antibiotic develops! The valuable medication goes to waste.'

'I ask patients who come from small towns about which medicines the general practitioner there has prescribed. They produce a whole collection of bottles. Most of these medicines are manufactured by small pharma companies. Obviously, these companies would have offered many inducements to these doctors to prescribe these medicines. Many of the doctors don't even have an MBBS degree. I don't think they know much about these medicines,' says Dr Suhas Bhave, a paediatrician from Sangli, Maharashtra.

Summing up ...

You might be feeling a shiver of apprehension after reading all of this. Maybe a certain sense of helplessness too. There is absolutely no doubt that it is high time to take the entire situation seriously, and to do something about it.

Chapter 4

Health Care Becomes an 'Industry':
The Growing Influence of Corporate and Multi-speciality Hospitals

INTRODUCTION

During the past twenty years, following liberalization policies, the growth of the IT industry and other factors, as well as disposable incomes among certain classes, have increased—though this is not the case across the social spectrum. As one doctor has said, Pune city, which should have fifty Sassoon Hospitals (public hospitals), has only one, although new corporate and multi-speciality hospitals are coming up daily. They are bright and glittering. In some ways, they are like shopping malls. Sometimes they have even been registered as so-called charity hospitals, but their only objective is profit. Partly because of their state-of-the-art equipment, but also because of a growing lack of choice, as older hospitals run by trusts or individuals close down, people are going to these hospitals. Such hospitals deliberately foster the impression that they provide high-quality services, which justifies their high costs of care.

There is another important aspect of such 'hospital-malls'. New technology costs lakhs and crores of rupees. If these machines are now indispensable for diagnosis, hospitals run by individual doctors are less able to compete. If the medical sector is left to the mercy of the market, and if the foundation of the whole business is profit, where will this take us?

Doctors themselves say that privatization and the underlying unbridled profit orientation are destroying the basic virtues of medical services at the very roots. Are we prepared to listen to them and do something?

Times are changing rapidly. In the past twenty years, under the influence of globalization, liberalization and privatization, the influence of the market has grown tremendously. Increasingly, medical services are no longer oriented around family doctors and personalized doctor–patient relationships; they have now largely become a commodity to be sold and purchased in the market. Just as shopping malls came up to sell groceries and consumer goods, corporate and large multi-speciality private hospitals arrived to sell medical services. The majority of these hospitals are not owned or run by doctors. Seeing the large profits to be made in the private medical sector, non-medical investors are pouring money into these private medical businesses to maximize returns on their investment. Among others, politicians, industrialists and stock market operators have poured billions of rupees into developing 'hospital-malls'. The important driving factor in the growth of these commercial enterprises is not the professionalism of doctors, but the expectation of returns on big money that is being poured into them.

Twenty years ago, there were hospitals set up and run by individual doctors; many still exist today. But now under the onslaught of corporate 'hospital-malls', they are often threatened with closure. Let us now see what our doctors have to say about large corporate, multi-speciality hospitals.

1. Unwanted Investigations, Procedures and Operations

A pathologist from a metropolitan city says, 'In corporate hospitals, each patient may be seen by multiple specialists. An orthopaedic is called because the hands and feet are aching; a neurologist for numbness in the hands. They come and look at the patient and their charges are added to the bill. Is it useful for multiple specialists to examine a patient? This question is never even asked.

'In many private medical colleges, the students only see a few patients, and even fewer from the poorest sections. How will they develop social sensitivity?'

'In corporate hospitals, investigations are not based on what the patient's illness is, and whether there is a need for specific investigations. Given any complaint, they produce a list of investigations that must be done,' notes Dr H.V. Sardesai, practising physician from Pune.

A surgeon from a metropolitan city observes, 'Totally unnecessary surgeries are being performed in corporate hospitals. During investigations, they may see a small stone in the gall bladder. It is not causing the patient any problems. But they scare the patient into going in for a surgery.

'I know of a case where the patient was charged Rs 1.5 lakh for an inguinal hernia surgery done by laparoscope (surgery for inguinal hernia is one of the simplest operations).'

'Asking about the rising corporate hospital sector is a question that needs no answer. It is not just rising, but is now firmly established. Government health services have been weakened due to government indifference, and that is why there is scope for corporate hospitals to prosper. Due to the entry of corporates, the order of priorities has changed. Now the doctors' priority is no longer the best interests of the patients, but the profit earned by the shareholders of the company,' says Dr Arjun Rajagopalan, a surgeon from Chennai.

2. BLATANT COMMERCIAL MARKETING BY CORPORATE HOSPITALS

A gynaecologist from a big city is of the opinion, 'People's sensitivities have become numbed due to certain corporate hospitals. Once bills in these hospitals started mounting up to Rs 10–20 lakh, people began to consider our bills of Rs 40,000–50,000 as trivial. These hospitals are like malls. Our society does not need them. Instead, all tertiary health care should be provided by the government.'

A skin specialist from a big city comments, 'Public relations officers of many corporate hospitals keep roaming around to visit doctors; they entice doctors to send patients (to their hospitals) by tempting them with cuts. Nearly everybody indulges in this practice. It must be legally banned.'

Another big-city doctor, a general surgeon, notes, 'Labour leaders at factories in our city are now in the pay of corporate hospitals. They agree to arrangements for the health care of workers to be covered by the employer at a particular corporate hospital. Now none of those 5000 workers comes to me. If they do come, they take some minor treatment and then go to the contracted corporate hospital. They have to, otherwise their medical expenses are not reimbursed by the employer.

'I said to one such leader, "You protest against malls set up by Reliance. But now when you join up with the corporates, what are we smaller hospitals supposed to do? Besides, these corporate hospitals charge bills of Rs 1 lakh and more, while the surgeon gets only Rs 4000 to 5000.'

A general practitioner from a small town offers more on the topic: 'Corporate hospitals often engage in marketing in a variety of ways. "Buy one, get one free", "Discount week" . . . full-page advertisements, mostly full of falsehoods. They throw parties for general practitioners, and they give them cuts. On top of this, they throw parties and supply liquor to keep politicians in their thrall. Some corporate and large hospitals admit bogus patients under the Rajiv Gandhi Health Scheme (a publicly funded health insurance scheme). They give the admitted person money, and plenty to eat and drink. They prepare records showing that an angioplasty or angiography has been done on that person, when actually nothing has been done. I wonder how the government comes out with such schemes, without first regulating private hospitals. Without regulation, the basic objectives of such schemes are lost, and they become mechanisms for corporate hospitals to loot public funds.'

'I feel that there is no humanism to be found in corporate hospitals. Small hospitals are being destroyed due to these corporates. This must stop. In small hospitals, there is at least the possibility that the doctor has not lost his basic sense of humanism. They wait for the patient to make the payment. They give concessions. None of this happens in corporate hospitals,' observes another general practitioner from a small town.

An ophthalmologist from a big city says, 'Corporate hospitals maintain everything five-star style, but forget about the patient. When the patient comes, they give him lemonade or tea. They advertise that they have the latest hi-tech optics shop. The patient melts because of the free lemonade, and he buys a pair of spectacles that have an actual value of Rs 200 or so, for Rs 3000–5000! The in-house optician is the main income avenue of corporate hospitals. Sometimes they offer a free check-up. The scheme has a 20-per-cent-off offer, just like in a mall. The whole atmosphere is designed to tempt.

'Corporates can implement government schemes and insurance schemes. We run small hospitals, our reimbursements are delayed, and we don't have the time to keep making trips back and forth to get our payment from the insurance company.

'Corporate hospitals vie for tie-ups with large public sector companies. And the officials are more than eager to oblige. These public enterprises give exorbitant reimbursement to their employees; Rs 5000 for just a pair of spectacles, of course made available from corporate hospitals. The big corporates in Mumbai draw in cases from all over Maharashtra. But junior trainee doctors operate on those cases! Further, often the quality of these corporate hospitals is not as good as they claim in their advertisements. When they do a cataract operation, they sometimes make money even on the lens. They charge a high amount of money for an expensive lens, but implant an average-quality lens.'

'If a patient goes with my referral note, he gets 30 to 40 per cent off on an MRI (because I do not take any commission). One patient forgot to take my note. He was charged the full amount, and a cut went to some third party,' says Dr Rajiv Dhamankar, practising paediatrician in Alibag, Maharashtra.

'Nowadays people want glamour and marketing. They have become used to the mall culture. The concept of "master check-ups" (packages of large number of tests, of which many may be unnecessary) has gotten into their heads. Now doctors who practise ethically and scientifically are looked upon with contempt, because they obviously can't afford this glitter. But people often don't know what they are getting into by going to corporate hospitals,' remarks an ophthalmologist from a metropolitan city.

3. COMMERCIAL DEMANDS AND TARGET-RELATED PRESSURES ON DOCTORS

'I am a senior doctor, and patients come to me because of my reputation. The Chief Administrative Officer (CEO) of my corporate hospital still doesn't have the courage to ask me questions. But recently a young doctor who had joined our department told me, "Sir, every month there is a meeting with the CEO. He asks me questions because instead of having a 40 per cent conversion rate for OPD-to-operative, as per the target, my conversion rate is just 10–15 per cent. (Conversion rate means out of the total number of patients seen by the doctor, the percentage which are advised to undergo surgery or procedures. Rational doctors try to keep this rate low, but profit-driven hospitals try to maximize the number of surgeries and procedures, even if they are unnecessary). He tells me that such a low conversion rate will not do and that unless I increase it, I will have to leave the hospital." This young doctor will certainly surrender one day.

To survive professionally, he will start doing the additional 20–25 per cent of additional procedures that are not required by medical logic. What choice does he have? After studying so much, if one is to apply this in work, then often there is no alternative but the corporate hospitals. It won't be possible for him during his lifetime to set up his own hospital, so he will work for the corporates. And each corporate hospital has such targets! There is no getting out of it,' a super-specialist from a metropolitan city elaborates.

A senior cardiologist from Kolkata, Dr Gautam Mistry says, 'I qualified in cardiology from PGI, Chandigarh. For the first nine months, I did a government job. But our government was using me to just treat patients with ordinary coughs and colds. Obviously, I had to leave the job. Then I joined a major hospital and worked there for seven years. I felt stifled there too. In order to benefit the hospital and meet its commercial needs, one has to do things like keeping patients in the hospital longer than necessary, and doing unnecessary investigations and procedures (including angioplasty) since there was pressure from the management of the hospital. My conscience began pricking me, and I left that hospital. Since the past nine to ten years, I only do a consulting practice. Heart patients have to take care for their entire lives, and they need a cardiologist who keeps an eye on them. That is what I do nowadays. I am happy. Initially I would feel sad that I am actually an ICU expert and can perform angioplasties. Now I cannot use those skills. (In one sense, that is a loss to society.) But rather than compromise on ethics, I prefer this compromise. And now I am realizing that if both the doctor and the patient would take proper care, very few heart patients will need to be admitted to the hospital, and even fewer would need angioplasties. Now people all over the world have the same experience, and the medical sector is taking serious note of the overdose of angioplasties and bypass operations.'

A physician from Pune, Dr Shyam Kagal also shares, 'In the past, I was attached to a certain hospital. The hospital management told me plainly that if I wanted to continue to be attached to the hospital, I would have to admit a certain minimum number of patients every month. I stopped admitting patients there, because I could not give such a guarantee. In the first place I will admit patients only when necessary, and when admitting a patient I will consider the patient's convenience in the choice of hospital.'

'I work in a department where the head is an internationally renowned and ethical senior doctor. Therefore, the management of our hospital never pressurized me with targets. I have certainly heard that this happens in some places. But I often feel sad that once I admit a patient, I have no control over their bill. At most, I can waive my entire fees and give a rebate of Rs 10,000–15,000 on his total bill of Rs 5 lakh!' says a super-specialist from a metropolitan city.

A urologist from a metropolitan city declares, 'After one year I left the corporate hospital. It is not possible for any doctor with a conscience to stay there.'

A nephrologist from a metropolitan city states, 'First the corporate hospitals pay you a fat salary. And then they put the responsibility of earning that salary back on the doctor. And if he can't manage it, then out with him. I know of things like unnecessary kidney biopsies being done under such pressure.

'A senior, super-specialist urologist I know left the corporate hospital. Because the young MBBS CEO was asking him why he had not performed a particular operation for removal of a kidney stone! There is no need for an operation for such a small stone which does not cause any problem. But the super-specialist did not have the right to take such a rational decision.'

'Earlier I too had left the corporate hospital. But then I rejoined when they begged me to come back and assured me I could practise on my own terms. They don't trouble me now. They need some well-known doctors around,' asserts a gynaecologist from a metropolitan city.

A surgeon from a metropolitan city states, 'In case a doctor feels that a patient will benefit by just spending two more days in hospital, he cannot do this in a corporate hospital. There he is questioned immediately. Just as a commercial airline does not make money unless the planes fly, corporates are not content unless there is some procedure or operation going on related to each bed in the hospital.

'I recently interviewed a young doctor. He was working in a super-speciality corporate hospital. Incessant targets, incessant pressure. First questioning, and then a kick on his backside if he does not meet his targets, whether by good means or bad. Fed up with this, he was willing to join us on a much reduced salary.

'In my own family, an insurance claim was rejected with the foolish remark that it was a pre-existing disease. Who decides this? On what basis? . . . There is no clear reason.'

Dr Jayant Das, a skin specialist from Kolkata, offers his point of view: 'New technologies come in. And then the new technology is dumped onto the patient as "the best treatment for the illness". For example, hair transplants, test-tube babies (IVF), and laser treatments. What is the success rate? What are the complications? There is no transparency about this. And there is a rush to try these treatments—which should be the last resort—before even trying other standard treatments, because crores of rupees have been invested by the hospital. Therefore, the rates are also very high. The patient is cheated into taking the treatment even where there is no need for it.'

'A corporate hospital invited me to join them. For a month, I pondered over the offer and finally I rejected it. By doing this, I lost a lot of potential income. But I am sure that in that money-making business, I would have had to look at patients solely from the perspective of increasing the hospital's profit. I am happier outside the corporate world,' a physician from a metropolitan city shares their experience.

'When one of my patients was doing a routine test, some changes were seen in the ECG. The patient had no complaints, but worried about the changes found in his ECG, he went to a famous cardiologist. The cardiologist performed an echocardiogram test. Even though this was normal, he then performed an angiography and advised angioplasty. Instead of getting an angioplasty performed, the patient came to me for a second opinion. I performed a repeat ECG, which came out as normal. He had no need of any treatment, let alone angioplasty! Such unnecessary procedures are advised because there is pressure on the cardiologist from the multi-speciality hospital to meet their targets,' notes Dr Partha Pritam Das, a general practitioner in Kolkata.

Dr Sanjay Gupte, a gynaecologist in Pune and former national president, FOGSI, says, 'Corporate hospitals want only those doctors who can help them earn more money. As a result, doctors who practise ethically cannot last there. I know of a hospital where if the patient is charged Rs 1,50,000, the doctor gets a mere Rs 15,000. Ninety per cent of the income goes into the corporate coffers.

'Corporate hospitals can advertise, while individual doctors are not allowed to do so! There are two types of advertisements. One is direct. And the other method is paid news! Now even the media admits that there is some such "paid news". The individual doctor sets up his clinic in some place. But he can't advertise and let people know about it! How are people to know that he has set up a practice? Should we permit him to advertise after setting some restrictions? It is something we need to think about.'

An ENT specialist from a big city adds, 'Presently the greatest danger is from insurance companies and corporates. Am I expected to take just Rs 5000 out of a bill of Rs 60,000 as offered by insurance companies for my surgery? Why should I slog for these insurance companies and corporates?

'The patient knows this. When a patient pays the insurance premium, it is his right that he should get the insurance cover. But what about me? When performing a surgery, I accept full legal responsibility. Not even 1 per cent of this responsibility is borne by the corporate or the insurance company. But just Rs 15,000 for me out of a bill of Rs 1,50,000? An insured patient came to my clinic and told me that he was voluntarily prepared to pay me additional fees. Because he felt that it was not proper that the insurance company would pay me so little, and so much to the corporates! This is the sorry state of affairs, when even the patient is moved to take pity on me. Now my beloved profession has gone to the dogs. I am totally dissatisfied.'

'There are a few exceptional corporate hospitals that work well. But usually, if you don't give the hospitals the income they want, they drive you away. They pay fat salaries, but they continuously dangle the sword of Damocles over you,' heeds paediatrician Dr Vandana Prasad in Delhi.

Dr Chandrakant Pandav, head of the Centre for Community Medicine at AIIMS, New Delhi discloses, 'There was a case in Delhi that was reported in the media. A psychiatrist was fired because she did not meet the hospital's target.'

4. Lack of Any Rules and Regulations, Negligent Treatment

A general practitioner from a small town says, 'These corporate hospitals are terrible. Hospitals run by individual doctors still have some remaining sense of humanism; those doctors who run the hospital have to deal directly with people. But corporate hospitals focus only on the cash.

'I'll tell you a true story. There was a death in a corporate hospital in the nearby city. A bill of Rs 16 lakh was prepared for a simple case of heart attack. The relatives didn't have the money. And so the corporate hospital hid the dead body! Finally the DSP had to raid the hospital. Such incidents are horrible.

'There's a family I know personally. The husband was about forty years old. He had a rare blood cancer, which the patient rarely survives. But the cancer specialist at the corporate hospital falsely assured the relatives that the chances of survival was 50 per cent, and told them that the expense of the treatment would be about Rs 4 lakh. His wife had a job which earns about 8000–9000 rupees a month. She set out to sell their two-room house to meet the treatment expenses. Hearing this, I could not restrain myself, so I went to meet her personally, though I had no connection with the case. I explained the matter to her and her relatives. Therefore, at least her home was saved. The husband was going to die anyway . . . and this woman and her children would have landed on the street!'

'When I see the charges at these corporate and multi-speciality hospitals, I start worrying about my old age,' comments a pathologist from a big city.

A big-city general surgeon informs, 'A gynaecologist put a stitch in a pregnant woman's uterus. Thereafter, probably due to the needle having mistakenly caused some damage to the membranes around the foetus, she began to drip fluid. Being worried, after a couple of days she went back to the gynaecologist. Her houseman removed the stitch and delivered the baby. But due to the earlier damage, she developed a severe infection. She was admitted to a corporate hospital, which performed a sonography every day. Every sonography report showed pus formation in her lower abdomen. That pus could have been immediately removed by just inserting a needle. But they were not doing anything. When I inquired, I came to know a shocking reality. That corporate hospital has a totally irrational rule: to charge double when the case enters the second week of admission and onwards. I'm sure that all this time-wasting was done in her case, so that they could charge the patient at double rates.'

A general surgeon from a medium-sized city shares, 'There is a BAMS doctor in our town who was my friend. His practice was very straightforward. Once his car hit lightly against a truck in front, which braked suddenly. The steering wheel mildly hit his chest and stomach. He drove the car onwards, and did not suffer any problems the whole day. Later, he suddenly broke out into a sweat and experienced chest pains. He was immediately taken to a multi-speciality hospital in a nearby city. An angiography and then an angioplasty were performed. The next day, he complained his stomach area was paining, but nobody in the ICU paid any attention. I reached that afternoon and was told about it. I immediately narrated the history of the blunt injury to my friend's chest and abdomen to the resident doctor of the ICU, and told him to promptly get an abdominal sonography done, and to show the report to his senior doctor. I came back, and on the third day, I got a call saying my friend was in serious condition. His blood pressure (BP) was way below normal, the pulse rate was very high and his abdomen appeared swollen.

'When I inquired about the sonography report, I was shocked. Despite my being a general surgeon, after the passage of sixteen hours of my categorical advice, the sonography I had ordered urgently had still not been performed. I angrily phoned the cardiac surgeon. He arrogantly said, "This is a serious complication resulting from the angioplasty." When I retorted angrily, he said, "Why are you creating a nuisance?" and grudgingly ordered the sonography.

'When the sonography was done, it came to light that there was 2 litres of blood accumulated in the abdomen! The patient was immediately transfused blood. But it was too late to perform surgery. My friend died. And besides this, the family was handed a bill of Rs 8 lakh.

'With some friends, I went to the hospital management and demanded to know why the advised sonography was not performed in time, though a general surgeon had recommended it. They just stuck to their guns . . . claiming there was no mistake. They even showed us the case papers. They were all filled in properly to cover up the mistake. The corporate hospital has regular, hired lawyers to defend them. My friend's wife refused to sue the hospital. All we could do was bring the bill down to Rs 4 lakh.

'People have a mistaken idea that one gets high-quality care in corporate and large multi-speciality hospitals. But what I have described reflects the actual state of affairs. In my individually run hospital, the entire responsibility for the admitted patient is squarely mine. Therefore, such mistakes do not happen.

'This hospital I mention is a very successful big hospital in a megacity. In such hospitals, the main problem is that no single doctor takes responsibility for the admitted patient. And then the big ego of city super-specialists! This surgeon from a small town . . . who is he to teach us?

'Such hospitals can sometimes prove very dangerous to patients, as illustrated by this case. And due to their money power and army of hired lawyers, even a doctor does not dare to drag such hospitals to court. The virus of profiteering has become tremendously powerful in the private medical sector.'

5. GOVERNMENT POLICIES, LACK OF REGULATION AND MEDICAL INSURANCE

Dr Jana of Shahid Hospital in Chhattisgarh shares, 'The government is shirking its responsibility. In Chhattisgarh, they have an agreement with certain corporate hospitals, without any regulation or control. In fact, in a majority of cases it is the corporate hospitals who decide who should be operated on. The government provides land to certain corporate hospitals nearly free of cost, with the condition that they should treat poor patients free of charge. But they don't take even one free patient. They project the patients for whom they get reimbursement from the health insurance schemes, as "free" patients on paper.

'In earlier days, doctors would set up their own hospitals. But now business-minded persons have entered the scene. They sell health care the way they sell slippers. They have no interest in medical ethics or in the values of the medical profession. A corporate hospital does business just like a shoe store. Tests and procedures are conducted in corporate hospitals—not because they are needed, but in order to make money for these hospitals.

'There is no structure for regulation of the charges; there is no logic to the charges. Whatever they feel like, they charge! In order to earn money, insurance companies will try to ensure that the lowest possible number of people get the lowest possible amount of treatment. In turn, private doctors will extract money from insurance companies. They will do admissions and operations even when there is no need.'

'Corporates and insurance companies are hand in glove in the matter of charges. If a corporate hospital charges Rs 75,000 for a delivery in Pune, and if the insurance company accepts it, what is one to make of the situation? I don't understand this mess. I'll give you my personal example. I had an angioplasty done in a corporate hospital in Mumbai. I was admitted at 10 a.m. and by 2 p.m. all the procedures were complete. They told me to pay Rs 4 lakh by that time. The corporate hospital did not give even a doctor like me concession of a single paisa. Cheques are not accepted. Neither are bank drafts. Just pay Rs 4 lakh in cash! Somehow or the other, I paid it within those four hours. This is not something the common man can do,' says Dr Rajendra Malose, a general practitioner from Chandwad in the Nasik district of Maharashtra.

A gastroenterologist from a metropolitan city observes, 'Nowadays the government engages private companies for its laboratory and radiology work. Under the public-private partnership agreement, there is a clause that BPL patients should be treated free of cost by the private partner. The proportion of BPL cases is very high in government hospitals . . . there are just a few who are not BPL. In such a situation, these private companies should not be making any profit. But they do. This obviously means that they refuse free treatment to many poor patients.

'This PPP policy of the government, which shirks its responsibility and enables corporates to make profits, should be stopped.

'The government has given free land to many large trust hospitals. As if this is not enough, due to their pressure, the customs duty on some imported machinery was reduced. Many of these trust hospitals practically run the business on the lines of corporate hospitals, and they have never offered the 10 per cent free and 10 per cent concessional services which they were supposed to do. The government should immediately cancel the licence of such hospitals.'

Private medical practice itself has some basic contradictions. The ideal situation would be when doctors do not engage in business by taking money from patients. Because, when considerations of their own benefit enter the business, doctors will be tempted to see how they can make more money while providing medical services. And the patient too will insist that if he is paying money, he should get the health care the way he demands. However, as many changes as you make in the system, it is not possible to entirely get rid of this contradiction. That is why we need to have a "universal health care" system, as in the UK.

'There is one benefit of corporate and multi-speciality hospitals. They cannot charge whatever amount they want. The charges are levied exactly as they have been fed into the computer. In hospitals run by individuals, charges are levied arbitrarily,' notes a super-specialist from a metropolitan city.

Another super-specialist from a metropolitan city recognizes, 'Some good things also happened due to the corporate sector. First, the quality of complicated tertiary services improved. Second, one can provide equipment here which individual doctors cannot afford to purchase on their own. Take robotic surgery—the robot costs Rs 10 crore. Nobody can possibly arrange for this at an individual level. New technologies certainly have their own importance and value, and we should not forget that corporate hospitals are now meeting this need.'

'In the central parts of the metropolis, there are many trust-run, service-oriented hospitals. Some are a hundred years old, but they are now being rapidly transformed into corporate hospitals; just as small theatres had to close down due to the advent of multiplexes. Is this the direction hospitals too are to take? It is a big issue,' says Dr Rajib Dasgupta, public health specialist at Jawaharlal Nehru University, Delhi.

Chapter 5

Social Attitudes and the Policy Context

The private medical sector in India today is completely unregulated. And now we have booming private medical colleges. A large proportion of private medical practitioners have BAMS and BHMS degrees, and have no systematic training in allopathy. Along with MBBS super-specialists, these general practitioners too have set up hospitals. Today, both these types of private hospitals mainly have earning money as their central focus. Over the past thirty years, the government has actively encouraged private medical colleges. There are other problems at the social level: lack of faith in doctors, propaganda against good doctors, the unrealistic attraction towards new medical technologies, and the fact that over the past twenty to thirty years health care has increasingly come to be viewed as a commodity for buying and selling. These changes driven by the market are associated with a trend towards 'medical consumerism' among many patients. Overall the situation is very anarchic. Both rational, ethical doctors and patients are being harmed by this situation. It is an urgent priority to find some solution. Otherwise, there is no saying where this degradation will lead us.

As mentioned earlier, the majority of the seventy-eight doctors who participated in this survey are engaged in a struggle to survive as ethical practitioners in an increasingly commercialized environment.

But they feel isolated. All these doctors complain that society does not support honest doctors! It is true that in the past twenty years the medical profession has been driven by privatization, market-promoting policies, growing consumerism and, above all, high profits. Common people are being swept away by this whirlwind. Government policies—for instance, state encouragement of private medical colleges—and social attitudes also contribute to doctors becoming like businessmen. But doctors must bear their due share of responsibility for the decline in ethical practice; patients too, and society as a whole colludes in this process of commercialization. And a system which tends to pit patients against doctors as buyer versus seller type adversaries in a market scenario is sharpening such conflicts.

Let us see how these doctors perceive society's role in the growing commercialization of medicine.

1. CHANGING SOCIAL ATTITUDES AND THEIR NEGATIVE INFLUENCE ON THE MEDICAL PROFESSION

Dr Vivek Sheth, an anaesthetist from Goregaon, Maharashtra, shares, 'I am an honest, experienced and reasonably competent doctor. If I am fearful of getting beaten up every time I work in a risky area like anaesthesia, don't you think there is some fundamental flaw in our system?

'We often make the mistake of judging all doctors on the same scale. The quacks and unqualified doctors, the traditional doctor who gives treatment as per his ancestral tradition, and the consultant with a valid degree in allopathic medicine—are they all "doctors"?

'In every town, we have some bogus gynaecologists who run nursing homes without any qualifications and training. They too are part of this syndrome. Their USP is: "We don't do caesareans, only normal deliveries, GUARANTEED! Isn't the acceptability these people have in society, particularly among educated people, a matter of concern?'

Dr Shyam Ashtekar, from Dindori, Nasik, says 'There is almost no chance that you will get patients if you engage in ethical practice. Even if you tell patients that a hysterectomy is not necessary, the majority of them will get it performed elsewhere. People cannot bear the thought of their patient dying, and so all costs keep rising. This must stop. However advanced science may be, however expert the doctor may be, however many procedures and investigations have been carried out—but in the field of medicine there is no guarantee that no patient will ever die, that we can diagnose the ailment immediately and cure it. This is an unavoidable boundary. Today society does not accept this. It is frightening that society today does not accept these boundaries. Because then commercial doctors and hospitals will exploit this attitude, and the doctor engaged in ethical practice will always feel the pressure of doing a test to confirm that a patient is not that one exception among a million. If one were not to do this test, and if things go wrong tomorrow, people will ask why the doctor did not do this procedure. For example, given a complaint of headache for a few days, should one just prescribe simple paracetamol tablets costing Rs 10, or should one recommend that the patient get his eyes tested, or should one do a CT scan? If the patient is going to blame me in the future if I do not do the scan, I will perform it today and put my cut in my pocket! Even those who practise honestly have become victims of society's unrealistic expectations.'

'IT professionals and those working in the corporate sector can be very rude. They don't want to wait their turn, and they casually ask for inflated bills, including bills for procedures that have not been performed. I wonder, "Even after earning so much, they are still greedy for more,"' adds a dentist from a metropolitan city.

A paediatrician from a metropolitan city mentions, 'Nowadays patients are just unable to understand the uncertainties of this profession. Why should one test for a disease that has a very low probability of occurring? One is fearful that patients may ask why the test was not performed. Nobody is willing to hear the line, "You don't need any medicine."'

'Don't reveal my identity. Because 90 per cent of the general practitioners today are BHMS or BAMS degree holders. They have political connections. They are already trying to get rid of me. My practice is now twenty-five years old. I charge just Rs 40 for an examination. I don't give even a single injection. I see 150 patients daily in my OPD clinic. Every day I get into conflict with these other doctors. My patients show me referral notes given by these commercial doctors recommending totally unnecessary surgeries. I tear up those notes and tell patients to go home! These doctors collectively suffer a daily loss of Rs 20,000–30,000 because of me. That is why they don't want me here. This is the horrendous reality. Will this change? I am determined not to give in. But another doctor might surrender out of fear, and I wouldn't blame him,' a general practitioner from a metropolitan city shares candidly.

Dr Medha Malose, from Chandwad, in the Nasik district, comments, 'Even when there is no need, people want hysterectomies and saline drips.'

Dr Rajendra Malose, a general practitioner from Chandwad in the Nasik district, also remarks, 'The patient is on a shopping spree. Just as tiled roofs on houses vanished over the past few decades, so did the doctor–patient relationship. Society has changed. Even in rural areas today they use the internet. Globalization, mobile phones . . . all these have a double-edged effect. How is it, that even a tribal woman comes to the clinic during pregnancy to find out whether she is going to have a boy or a girl? Doctors have converted patients into commodities. Today's young general practitioners understand the process of commercialization. They conduct camps and perform unindicated hysterectomies. I might say with a little exaggeration that nowadays one rarely sees a woman over the age of 35–40 years who still has her uterus. The PCPNDT law (prohibiting sex-determination tests through sonography) has often been used by bureaucrats to harass good doctors. I too closed my medical termination of pregnancy (abortion) centre to avoid the hassle. I returned the sonography machine. Enough! After thirty years of honest practice oriented towards the poor, if they are going to harass us rather than the crooks, let people go 70 km away to have a sonography.

'Many people come to us to get insurance benefits by filling in false papers. I am the only doctor who refuses. The rest give in.'

A paediatrician from Delhi, Dr Vandana Prasad says, 'Due to pressure put by patients, even my own prescriptions for cough syrup increased. Patients are not willing to accept that I don't give any medicine.'

'Due to insurance, patients feel that they should get treatment in a five-star hospital. They don't care about what the quality of treatment is,' says Dr Satish Gosain, a general practitioner from Delhi, of his own experience.

On the subject of insurance, Dr Sanjay Bhatnagar, a paediatrician in Delhi, mentions, 'Having taken insurance, a patient feels like a king. The patient casually uses the insurance card like a debit card. They ask me, "Can you get me admitted and help me earn some money?" I refuse. But I know of some hospitals where they don't actually admit patients, but merely prepare the paperwork. The hospital, the patient and the TPA (Third Party Administrator) share the proceeds among themselves.'

A renowned physician from Pune, Dr H.V. Sardesai says, 'The overall level of ethical behaviour in our society has declined. There is a shortage of honesty. Doctors too often have a lack of ethics. One of the reasons for this is also that if a doctor has a Mercedes, society considers him great.

'The patient does not change his own lifestyle. Doctors should be able to tell such patients that if he doesn't obey instructions, then he won't get medicine. But this does not happen.'

Another physician from a metropolitan city adds, 'Now patients fall prey to the marketing of master check-ups and undergo many unnecessary tests. They then get worried over minor problems in some test results, and come to the doctor, not because they have some genuine problem! This is tantamount to putting the cart before the horse. Totally unnecessary but alluring diagnostic tests, their marketing and the patient who falls prey to the marketing—this is today's reality.'

Dr George Mathai, a physician from Alibag, Maharashtra, acknowledges, 'Patients' expectations too have become unrealistic. In a few cases, rare ailments may not get diagnosed. Then the patient asks why a particular test had not been performed. There are only a few such patients, but the increased expectation creates problems and the patients have begun to ask for monetary compensation from the doctors. This kind of monetary compensation under tort law is not suited to any society or medical system. Only lawyers earn in such a system. As a result of such trends, there is a horrible problem in the US. It is not good that we are repeating the error.'

A gynaecologist from Pune, Dr Pratibha Kulkarni recognizes, 'The perspective from which society views doctors is changing. It may be because of doctors' own misdeeds, but nowadays patients look upon doctors with suspicion. Up to a certain point, the patient should definitely ask questions. Doctors must of course be accountable. But sometimes patients and their relatives behave in an unreasonable manner. Just a few days ago, a well-educated young woman came here. I had treated her sister successfully, and she was now pregnant. This girl created a scene in front of the other patients. When this patient had undergone a sonography in her twentieth week, no abnormality had been detected in her foetus. But in the twenty-fifth week, the sonography showed a defect in the kidney. This girl was aggressively quarrelling with us, asking how we had made such a mistake earlier. I kept telling her that kidney and heart defects cannot be seen during the twentieth week, but only around the twenty-fifth week. But she wouldn't listen. Now what is to be done?'

As an aside, a gynaecologist from a big city comments, 'People don't want to accept nowadays that apart from the doctor they too have a responsibility towards their health. They don't want to make efforts for any dieting or exercise. Some of them blatantly tell lies.'

'A baby was brought to the clinic. There was nothing wrong with the baby, and I said that there is no need for any medicine. It is just gas in the tummy, go home. And then, the same evening, I get a call from a general practitioner saying that he is sending a baby for serious treatment. It was the same baby. The diagnosis from the sonography mentioned that the baby has a twisted intestine. Actually the baby was fine; it was laughing and playing. I admitted the baby and just watched it. The next day I sent the baby home. That patient had of his own accord done a sonography, when there was no need for it,' shares Dr Rajiv Dhamankar, a paediatrician from Alibag, Maharashtra.

A gynaecologist from Pune, Dr Pratibha Kulkarni, mentions, 'Nowadays people have more faith in technology and in printed reports than in my clinical knowledge. One young woman who was pregnant came to me with a sonography report showing that there was inadequate fluid in her uterus. I examined her and assured her that there was no problem; everything was fine. She would not believe me. She went to a big hospital with that report. There they admitted her for a fortnight! She was given a saline drip with so-called medicines that are of no use. Of course her report was not going to change. Then she came back to me.'

2. Lack of Appropriate Policy/Harassment by the Government Machinery

An ophthalmologist from a medium-sized city offers, 'In many towns and cities, BAMS, MD Ayurvedic degree holders in gynaecology and ophthalmology are now performing operations. What kind of government regulation is there to check this? Can doctors perform such surgeries with just a BAMS (basic Ayurvedic) degree? How can they use allopathic medicines when they want to? The patients are not informed about the scope and limitations of these degrees.

'Cheating and confusion in surgeries has become today's reality. In our society there is no knowledge about various degrees, and there is no shortage of doctors with such degrees. Due to blind belief, that whoever calls himself a doctor has a magic hand to cure, anarchy prevails.

'It is quite disturbing to see such shortcut MD Ayurvedic doctors being allowed to perform operations without any restrictions. It is very frustrating for genuine specialist doctors.'

An ophthalmologist from a big city shares, 'Those who have graduated from private medical universities and those with diplomas that are not recognized by the MCI, create chaos in medical practice. They hardly know anything. This must stop. Those people who set up hospitals worth Rs 40 crore nowadays have come there after spending Rs 1 crore on donations in a private medical university. All they are concerned about is how they can make Rs 40–80 crore in the first year.'

A pathologist from a big city mentions, 'Our politicians and policymakers have permitted colleges offering DMLT (Diploma in Medical Laboratory Technology) pathology degrees to be opened in every lane. I am told, "These technicians' colleges just take money and give degrees. They don't teach anything." Even consultants send their patients to them for test reports because they get 60–70 per cent commission from these technicians. I know a technician who has been using the wrong bulb for measuring blood sugar for the past twenty-five years. Over the last twelve years I have myself seen this technician miss eight to ten cases of blood cancer. I feel sad that even my MBBS friends—though they have now become consultants—do not send me patients because I do not give cuts. Some of them even appoint such technicians in their hospitals and earn money themselves on pathology reports. It is difficult to understand to what extent this is going to go.'

A practising gynaecologist in Pune, Dr Pratibha Kulkarni also shares, 'Here, almost 50 per cent of deliveries are done by caesarean operation. It is true that doctors often perform caesareans when not required—but now the patients are crucial participants in this process. Just a few days ago, I was giving a trial of normal delivery to a patient. It was a difficult case. But I was trying my best to ensure that it was done normally, without an operation. But something that happens often nowadays took place. Her father came and said, "Look, doctor, perform a caesarean if necessary. There should be no unnecessary risk to the mother and the baby."

'I asked, "Who told you that there is no risk in a caesarean? It is true that the risks of caesareans have reduced considerably since the development of good-quality suturing material and antibiotics. But that does not mean that caesareans have become lower-risk than normal deliveries."

'But who is there to convince those who pressurize doctors to perform caesareans?

'And how is any gynaecologist to resist this pressure? And nowadays, everybody feels that since they are paying money, there should be no complication. Nobody is ready to accept the uncertainty that is part of the medical profession. Even in our hospital, if there is an unexpected death, people resort to violence. Doctors are forced to live under protection!'

'The present government systems create problems for everyone. New laws torment doctors and in my opinion they achieve nothing much apart from this. My friends and I have now been practising for fifteen years. Many of my friends have left India and have migrated abroad. The frightening truth is that honest doctors will not be able to survive at an individual level. Laws are being prepared with the influence of corporates, and society does not do anything. One feels sad, insecure. The direction that has been taken is making smaller hospitals unable to function,' offers an ENT specialist from a metropolitan city.

Dr Jayant Das, a skin specialist from Kolkata, acknowledges, 'There has been a remarkable decline in the quality of medical education. In government colleges, good teachers feel suffocated and denigrated due to hierarchical and bureaucratic ways of functioning. The atmosphere is not at all encouraging. And due to this, the doctors who graduate have no self-confidence. Given this lack, and the other inducements on offer, these young doctors quickly fall prey to tendencies for irrational care.'

'All regulatory bodies are harassing doctors. Many laws are coming in. I am not opposed to the laws but their implementation is such that it harasses each doctor,' comments Dr Sanjay Gupte, a gynaecologist and ex-president of FOGSI in Pune.

3. The Harmful Influence of Private Medical Colleges—Boon or Bane?

A general surgeon from a metropolitan city states, 'I am associated with a private medical college. Actually, when I was a resident, the organization MARD (an association of resident doctors) had gone on strike when the first private medical college was opened. The government broke our strike. Some doctors went to court, but the court silenced them by raising some technical issues. One is saddened by the fact that our society does not see what is happening. Those who take admission into private medical colleges pay lakhs of rupees. It appears that they have no knowledge about the quality of the college. There is indifference all around.

'The reality is horrible. The majority of these colleges belong to politicians. They are being run from a business perspective. All they focus on is where they can make more money and where they can save money. These people give grand speeches but they are nothing but hardcore businessmen. The result is that students are not allowed to go to the operation theatre, as one needs to arrange separate clothes for them, and these colleges save money by cutting such expenses. Besides, there is always a frantic effort to get the maximum number of postgraduate seats.

'The result is that no student is failed; a student will fail only if he falls at your feet and begs, "Please fail me." Like grocers, they maintain two separate books of accounts. One is to show the MCI and one is for themselves. And interns are placed in the Medical Records Department. They write up bogus cases. Nobody is concerned even about the fact that right from the beginning of their working lives these doctors are taught to see such fraud as "normal business". Everything is frightening. Even if this reality is exposed, the power of the politicians is such that no action will be taken.

'The biggest wonder is what they examine during an inspection. I am sure that they would be satisfied even if they get a NAAC degree (National Assessment and Accreditation Council) with "D" grade. But they get a "B". It's amazing. You can imagine how they got this grade. Students will see this grade, and pay money to come to this college.

'We have sunk to such depths that I have come to the conclusion that things will improve simply because there is no way that they can become worse.'

Another surgeon, Dr Arjun Rajagopalan from Chennai, remarks, 'Out of more than forty medical colleges in Tamil Nadu, half are private. I have heard that a seat in radiology (sonography/MRI) costs Rs 4 crore. An ordinary MBBS seat costs Rs 65 lakh. One sees no authority effectively regulating these colleges.'

'Nowadays the practice of putting a stitch at the mouth of the uterus has increased a lot. There is an important reason for this: this is what is taught in certain private medical colleges. In these colleges, students only learn how to read a sonography report, not how to examine a patient. In a private medical college, 20–25 caesareans take place in a month. There are only three to four normal deliveries. These doctors have little knowledge about normal deliveries. They quickly get scared and perform a caesarean,' adds a gynaecologist from a big city.

Another gynaecologist from a big city shares, 'What can I tell you? Just a few days ago a fresh MD called me. He had done his MD from a private college. It was a posh hospital. A woman from the trading community came to his private hospital for the first time. She wanted an abortion. It was done. She went home. She returned after a week because her bleeding and stomach ache did not stop. This MD performed a sonography. One can see the clear diagnosis that some matter has remained in the uterus.

'What would I have done? This can happen to anybody. I would have explained to the patient and immediately done a curetting (minor procedure to clean inside the uterus). End of the matter.

'But this fellow just kept giving her antibiotics and tablets. A sonography every two days. The same diagnosis in every sonography. Higher antibiotics.

'After a few days, it turned septic. Fever, BP, pulse: everything was alarming.

'He called me. He said. "The patient has septicaemia (severe infection that has spread to the bloodstream). We may have to remove the uterus."

'I replied, "You should at least have called me earlier." He retorted, "I'm calling you now, aren't I?"

'First, this inadequate experience and on top of that this arrogance.

'Even after twenty years of practice, when I have a doubt I take a second opinion from a senior. Our generation respected seniors. Now they look upon them with contempt.

'And at the end it is the patient who suffers.

'Extremely rude. Drunk with the power of money. One is saddened.'

Dr Jana, from Shahid Hospital in Chhattisgarh, adds, 'Clinical practice and its associated skills are now dying out.'

Dr H.V. Sardesai, practising physician in Pune, comments, 'Admissions to medical colleges should be strictly on merit, not on the basis of money.'

'What is one to expect from a boy who has paid a crore or two for admission? Private medical colleges are a monster, just like pharmaceutical companies,' remarks Dr Rajendra Malose, a general practitioner from Chandwad, Maharashtra.

4. Issues Revealed in Some Informal Conversations

Arun Gadre has practised medicine for more than twenty years. He notes: Over the past eight years, I have been travelling all over Maharashtra. Wherever I go, I naturally have some doctor friends and we chat. Here below I have given some of the observations that I have noted down from these conversations:

- The Supreme Court made it legally compulsory to implement certain fire safety measures. In some medium-sized cities there is no mechanism that can certify this. It's all confusion. Then how is the registration to be renewed? A way out has been found by taking written assurances from the doctors that they would implement those measures, but doctors have been forced to make some 'significant' compromises to operationalize this solution.

- In one city, it has been made compulsory by officials to purchase fire safety equipment from one particular company. Obviously, the person who sells this equipment is a relative of a concerned government official.

- There is an expectation of a 'meaningful' contribution to the sarkari babu when one renews one's registration for sonography.

- In case a patient dies in the hospital and the body has to be sent for a post-mortem, we soon get a phone call from the government doctor performing the post-mortem: 'Is there anything to be altered to safeguard your interest?' And in case we say no, threatening comments are made: 'We will give a damning report against you.' So in reality, even if the doctor has not committed any error but he or she does not give a bribe, there is a possibility that a false indicting report is given for post-mortem because one of the officers in government hospitals who performs the post-mortem is corrupt.

- Many people know juicy and amazing tales about the inspections of private medical colleges, such as hiring doctors and patients for just a day, to appear before the inspection team, and similar stories.

- Without any compunction, many doctors engaged by private medical colleges sit at home and collect their salaries from the college. They go once in two months and sign in. But they are shown on the muster of the college as fulfilling legal requirements.

- Nowadays, politicians consider a death in a hospital an opportunity to capitalize on, in order to make some money. The workers of these politicians turn up, and even if the doctor is not at fault, he is threatened. Some money is given to the relatives of the dead person, and the politicians and their workers end up earning well. 'We are not at fault. A patient can die in hospital or during surgery. Why then should we give in to such extortion?' doctors ask. Shrugging aside such reservations from honest doctors, big multi-speciality and corporate hospitals engage in such compromises. In this whole process, an honest doctor's self-respect is hurt, his confidence declines, and he loses joy in his work. The insurance companies, with which the doctor has taken an insurance policy to protect himself, also keep pressurizing the doctor in favour of such out-of-court settlements.

- Some individual doctors also keep aside money from their turnover for such 'settlements'. They give some money to end matters in cases where there have been complications or deaths, even when there have been no mistakes made by the doctor. Due to such distribution of money by some doctors, there is now an expectation in society that one should ask for money when there are complications or deaths in hospitals.

- Local politicians take advantage of these attitudes which have spread throughout society. In the midst of all this, it is the doctors who practise ethically that feel trapped. They feel very insecure. The result has been that these ethical and capable doctors, who would earlier take risks, have now started referring their patients to corporate and multi-speciality hospitals.

• Due to all this, patients may be in danger because they may not get timely treatment and may get care only after time-consuming referrals. Also, the treatment has become many times more expensive.

Summing up . . .

Doctors are moulded by the society in which they practise. Their value systems are shaped by that society as well. Unfortunately, widespread corruption is a common reality in India today and when doctors turn into entrepreneurs they have to confront this. For instance, while genuine regulation to promote standards of care and to protect patients is essential, regrettably unscrupulous officials can use these rules to harass doctors rather than safeguard patients' rights. The doctor–patient relationship has also come under stress, especially in situations where excessive commercialization has led to the connection becoming akin to a supplier–consumer tie. The doctors we interviewed were genuinely dismayed by this state of affairs. Our hope is that we can move from a commercialized, market-driven health care system, towards a socially regulated and publicly organized system, where maximizing profits is not the only concern. Otherwise, even the dwindling species of rationally practising and ethical doctors may be forced towards extinction. As Brecht has said, 'No one can be good for long, if goodness is not in demand.'

Chapter 6

Some Solutions Suggested by Doctors

Why have we converted health care into a commodity dictated by the market? Has this happened as a result of deliberate policy, or has this emerged as a default option due to 'policy blindness'? First, doctors were given a free hand to sell medical care as a service, and then people were dragged into accepting that there was not much choice but to purchase it. While we go into such analysis, the question remains: What solutions and remedies can we implement as a society? What will the social demands be?

Before we do this, let us see what the doctors in our interviews have to say about this. From their experience, these doctors are also saying some things about the cure for this social disease, although many are quite pessimistic about the possibility of change, as we can see from a few statements.

A general practitioner from Delhi, Dr Satish Gosain openly remarks, 'There is no solution to this mess.'

Dr Pratibha Kulkarni, practising gynaecologist in Pune, adds, 'I have so many questions, but can't think of any solutions. Are we to be satisfied just with the fact that we practise ethically? That's good. But this must improve.'

Nevertheless, there are a range of possible solutions that have been suggested by many of the doctors, which can be broadly categorized into: regulation of the private medical sector, strengthening public health services, developing doctor-patient dialogue forums and moving towards a system of universal health care.

1. SOCIAL REGULATION OF THE PRIVATE MEDICAL SECTOR, RATE STRUCTURE AND STANDARD TREATMENT GUIDELINES

Dr Arjun Rajagopalan, a surgeon from Chennai, says, 'Doctors engaged in private practice are being suffocated nowadays and having to shut shop. When I see this, I am very disappointed. Good people are being driven out. There is no means by which doctors can have an ethical practice. One sees the pharmaceutical companies and corporate hospitals throttling those who are ethical. I am saddened by this, and have more or less given up hope. Where will all this end? I don't know. Even sixty years after Independence, there is no system for effective supervision and regulation of the medical sector. The MCI has proven to be useless. Some of the corruption there has come to light in newspapers. The private medical sector needs to be brought under strict and effective regulation. There should be a review every year. This is very difficult. And one doesn't see anybody demanding this. There is no political will.'

An ophthalmologist from a big city adds, 'There is a dire need for a regulatory body. Allopathy and all other forms of medicine should be regulated. Treatment guidelines should be provided. Even if you permit BAMS and BHMS doctors to practise allopathy, certain boundaries need to be clearly laid down. These doctors just copy what we do. A rate structure also needs to be drawn up for all private doctors. Not only should treatment guidelines be prepared but there should be monitoring to ensure that they are followed.'

A pathologist in Pune, Dr Mandar Paranjpe mentions, 'Mechanisms like NABL (National Accreditation Board for Testing and Calibration Laboratories) to maintain quality are coming in. Actually, I already do 80 per cent of the things specified in these guidelines. But the standards suggested for location/ space of the laboratory are unrealistic.

'Further, the condition that a control test be conducted after a certain number of tests as a quality check is one that Indian patients cannot afford.

'Corporate hospitals can follow all these rules. But their rates are beyond the reach of the common man. Experts in India should sit together and find a practical solution.'

A radiologist from a big city comments, 'I have no problem with the PCPNDT (Pre-Conception Pre-Natal Diagnostic Techniques Act)—the act for preventing sex-selected abortion. I don't have to give a single paisa to the official who comes for the monthly monitoring. Often, I stay up late at night to fill in the paperwork. This law is appropriate. It has created fear. Such a law should be brought in for all regulation of all private medical practice. That will be very helpful.'

A general surgeon from a big city adds, 'Rates should be transparent. Through the Surgical Society, we are working towards standardization of rates. There is a need for regulation. But we should not implement American standards here. Do not forget that our doctors are better clinicians. You don't copy Western systems which could not be implemented. Then how can you force people to comply?'

A practising surgeon in a megacity states:

'The following improvements will have to be done on a priority basis:

1. Medical college admissions (including private medical colleges) should be made completely transparent. They should be done through entrance exams like the IITs.

2. Private medical colleges may charge fees similar to an MBA course, but there should be a heavy penalty for capitation fees.

3. The norms for setting up medical colleges should be changed. When more colleges come up, the capitation fee will reduce.

4. Fundamental changes need to be made in the medical curriculum, which have not been looked into for many years.

5. A new Medical Council Act: The Council presently has 123 members. The number of government bureaucrats among them needs to be reduced. There must be some patients' representatives in the Council.'

Pune-based physician Dr H.V. Sardesai offers, 'How many CT scans do you think there are just in Pune? Shouldn't there be a central agency that decides how many CT scans there should be in Pune? This is one important issue. But there is no agency and no control. What is happening is that a lot of CT scan machines are being installed. Then all kinds of malpractices are indulged in to attract patients.

'How is change possible? It is possible. It is possible to prepare a rate structure for all routine admissions, procedures and surgeries. There may be at most a discrepancy of 5 or 10 per cent.

'A law must be passed that only generic medicines may be prescribed.'

A general practitioner from a metropolitan city remarks, 'Depending on the area to be covered and the population, there should be designated general practitioners, specialists and facilities for investigations. Patients should not be allowed to go directly to the specialists. General practitioners should have strict protocols. A similar system is in place in the UK. One cannot just set up a clinic/speciality clinic or CT scan etc., wherever one desires. The number is restricted as per demographic and epidemiological need. There is a gatekeeper approach. One cannot jump the ladder and bypass the GP and approach a specialist. The GP has to refer the case to a specialist. This will go a long way to curb malpractices. Investigations should take place strictly according to those protocols. Send patients to the specialists only if needed.'

'The poor suffer since they don't have money for care. They do whatever they can to pay for the expenses. There should be a system whereby genuine BPL patients (there are many bogus cases among them) should get concessions in the private medical sector,' adds a skin specialist from a big city.

2. Strengthening Public Health Services, Promoting Genuinely Charitable Hospitals

Dr George Mathai, a physician in the Alibag district of Raigad, is of the opinion, 'The best model is that of genuine trust hospitals. This means that the trusts should build the hospitals so that the cost of construction does not have to be borne by patients. Private doctors should have attachments to these hospitals. A big financial burden will be over. It will be easier to monitor.

'Good government hospitals are the best means of keeping private practitioners in control. In Kerala, the rate charged by private practitioners is lower due to a better public health system. But thirty-eight years ago, when I was working full-time in a civil hospital in Maharashtra, I was harassed by many of my colleagues because I was not part of the system of corruption. Nowadays things have become even worse.

'Trust hospitals are supposed to admit 10 per cent and 20 per cent patients free and at concessional rates respectively. We should be informed daily as to how many such beds are available in each hospital. Why is the internet not used for such things?'

A general practitioner in a rural area shares, 'Health care is a fundamental right of every citizen. The government services in rural areas and in civil hospitals have collapsed. Nowadays, a poor person has to sell all his belongings and go to a private hospital. Or else he must die quietly. When three or four persons from a family are in an accident, the whole family is destroyed. Let BAMS/BHMS doctors learn allopathy through a one-year course. Then appoint him to a sub-centre which services five villages and the government should pay him a salary. Give him permission and medicines to cure common ailments. People will do this happily. Get him to accept the condition, appoint him and give him a one-year course. If a patient wants any further treatment he must come with a referral note from this doctor or else he will not get further treatment. This will be an excellent mechanism.'

Public health expert, Dr Rajib Dasgupta at JNU, Delhi, comments, 'Over the past fifteen years, in the Delhi metropolitan area and in its surrounding areas, the Municipal Corporation built a number of medium-sized hospitals in a well-planned manner. There are, of course, some deficiencies in their functioning. They face a big problem of manpower and there is doubtless scope for improvement. But at least there is some scope for improvement because these hospitals actually exist now. Keep in mind that in the past the Municipal Corporation Hospital was only in the centre of the metropolis. Now these hospitals have been built in areas inhabited by the poor and lower middle classes. This is the direction in which change must take place. The government health services must be strengthened.

'In West Bengal, there is a town with a population of 2–3 lakhs. For twenty years, there was a government maternity home in the town which was limping along. A paediatrician was elected as the mayor and a retired school principal was elected as the deputy mayor. The two of them increased the municipality's expenditure on this hospital. The local MP helped them. Now it has 100 beds. The hospital has been attached to a medical college. All specialists are paid fees to come there and they do come. Now the municipality is making plans to make the hospital bigger. All the beds are always full.

'It is not as if there is a lot of poverty all around or that private medical services are not available. This is quite a prosperous town. Cash crops grow in the area; there is also a mine. There were plenty of private doctors there for many years. Doctors from outside would deliberately ask for transfers to this town because it was easy to get established, leave the job and set up a private practice. But this remarkable policy was formulated by the municipality and as a result, the 100 beds are always full. This means that private practice in the town has suffered.

'This is an important example. If politicians and those who work in the government system have the will, government health services can become very efficient. But we need to keep in mind that it is of no use just to increase government services in the form in which they currently exist. They need to grow with new concepts and new policies. They need to be efficient.'

3. Doctor–Patient Dialogue Forum

Dr Sanjay Gupte, gynaecologist and ex-President, FOGSI, Pune, discusses, 'The responsibility for the anarchy that we see today has to be borne, in descending order of importance, by the system, the individual doctor and, last of all, the patients. Improvements too will have to be made in the same order. It is essential that there be an improvement at all levels: in government systems, policies, the Medical Council of India and in the medical colleges. There is no regulation of private medical practice today—that will have to be introduced.

'Will it be possible to create such a forum? It can become feasible when civil society organizations get together with doctors who practice ethically in the city in different branches of medicine and open a dialogue with the patients. Patients' queries can be answered and second opinions can be given. If some such process begins to operate once a month, then there will be a moral pressure on all doctors. Patients will be reassured by the transparently given advice. It is essential that such a dialogue between doctors and patients takes place.

A super-specialist from a metropolitan city adds, 'There is a need to create a forum in which patients have faith. Treatment protocols have to be created and they must be strictly implemented. Then this forum, which will be composed of ethical doctors, will be able to explain the treatment protocols to patients. Thereafter, the pressure on doctors to order unnecessary investigations will reduce.

And if a doctor is not working properly and ordering unnecessary investigations he can be pulled up.'

4. MOVING TOWARDS UNIVERSAL HEALTH CARE

Pune-based physician Dr H.V. Sardesai remarks, 'There is a universal health care system in England. When undergoing any type of treatment, no money has to be paid by the patient. The payment is made by an autonomous body and the funds for this come from taxes. This is an ideal direction in which to move. We must make the effort. The medical profession needs to be separated from commercial considerations.'

Dr George Thomas, an orthopaedic surgeon in Chennai, also comments, 'In India, people have to select their doctor. This is not a good system. What knowledge do people have to enable them to make this decision? None. Then they decide which doctor to consult based on hearsay, or on information given by their relatives or friends. Now one even sees advertisements by private hospitals. How true are they? Nobody knows.

'If the decision is left to me, I would put an end to private practice in India. I am a doctor who got into private practice against my will. Before I die, my fervent hope and desire is to see a system like in England, which gives "free medical services to all"; a "Universal Health System" being set up in India.'

On the same topic, a physician from a big city discusses, 'If one doesn't bring in regulation by law, it will not be possible to implement mere guidelines.

'I have friends in the UK. One is an ENT specialist. But he is working in the UK as a general practitioner, and still, he is happy. The system in place there is very good. Such a system needs to be brought in here as well. Of course there are certain problems with the model. The main deficiency is that you do not get an early appointment if you have an ordinary illness.

'A patient from Germany was telling me that the doctors cannot spare even two or three minutes per patient. Social insurance exists there as well. But compared to the anarchy we have here, we have no alternative but to put in place a system like in the UK, after reducing its deficiencies.

'Yes, standard guidelines are possible. Actually, they are available on the internet. Who says that it is impossible? From the general practitioner to the super-specialist, every single doctor should have a manual containing these guidelines. After how many days should one call the patient back for an examination? How many days after changing the medication should one examine the patient again? There are guidelines even at this micro-level, and they are needed.

'I know for certain that any system is bound to fail in India because social conscience in India has reached its nadir. Dishonesty has become so firmly rooted in every pore of society that any improvement is impossible. Shouldn't the Medical Council of India monitor all these things? Corruption has struck deep roots everywhere. I read about it in the papers. Everything has become disgusting. In such a situation, where does one find the political and social will and, most important of all, minimum ethical values to make any improvement? I see no light at the end of the tunnel.'

'We definitely need to bring in a medical-services system in India, wherein there will be no direct financial dealings between doctor and patient. As long as money is paid and accepted, doctors will be tempted to engage in unethical practices. Universal Health Care (UHC) is such a system, and it is being implemented in around 40 per cent of countries globally. If it can be implemented in a country like Sri Lanka, which is poorer than India, why has it not been introduced in our country?' says Dr Punyabrata Goon, a general physician from Kolkata.

Dr Sanjib Mukhopadhyay, a gynaecologist from Kolkata, shares, 'I am now tired of arguing and quarrelling. There is a story in the Ramayana. Ravan abducted Sita. Grief-stricken, Rama and Laxman were searching for her in the forests. A tired Rama decides to have a bath in a pond. Before entering the water, he sticks his arrow's tip into the ground and leaves the arrow standing upright. After his bath, when he comes back, he sees that a frog crushed by his arrow's tip is on the verge of death.

'He asks the frog, "Oh, frog, when I was about to put my arrow into the ground, you should have called out!"

'The frog put his hands together and said, "Oh, Lord! I have been hearing that Lord Rama is a person who will do the world good. But when your arrow takes my life, I accepted defeat. If the one who is supposed to look after my welfare sets out to kill me, to whom can I complain?"

'With folded hands, I implore the government and doctors, "If you are going to shirk the responsibility of looking after the health of millions of poor people, who can save them?"'

Part Two:

Initiating the Cure

Chapter 7

Physicians, Heal Thy System!

We conducted interviews with seventy-eight doctors across the country, and have presented to the reader the key points emerging from this process in the preceding pages. Malpractices in private hospitals, the problematic impact of profit-driven corporate hospitals on the medical profession, the toxic influence of pharmaceutical companies, society's changing expectations, the role of government policies in the context of growing commercialization of medical services, and what directions these doctors see as a way out of the current situation—observations and opinions of the doctors on all these issues have been noted.

The reality of the private medical sector that becomes apparent through the prism of these reflections is painful and deeply disturbing. All these interviews underline the reality that the unregulated, highly commercialized and anarchic manner in which the private medical sector is operating today, is posing certain serious problems not only for society, but also for those honest doctors in the private sector who try to run their practice on ethical lines.

If this is the frightening reality today, what will be the situation in the next one or two decades? Is there a need for some urgent and far-reaching policy changes? This is something that citizens, civil society organizations, experts working in the health sector, organizations and groups of medical professionals, policymakers and of course, in our democracy, the government and politicians need to consider on a priority basis.

In any process of cure, the first step is properly understanding the disease. Regarding the private medical sector, we have taken one step in that direction through interviewing these doctors. These reflective doctors have skilfully diagnosed the extremely serious illnesses from which the private medical sector is suffering. Now we have to move from diagnosis to treatment, however difficult this may be.

What do these interviews with the doctors tell us? With the exception of a few doctors, the vast majority of interviewed doctors agree on the following points. These points are important, since they could form the basis for developing a consensus around an agenda for change, involving both rational doctors within the health care profession, and various kinds of citizens' groups and social movements.

1. The practice of giving commissions or cuts, as well as unnecessary investigations, procedures, treatments and surgeries have spread throughout the private medical sector. These are now the norm rather than exceptions; it is not as if only a few hospitals engage in such practices.

2. All the doctors agree that the influence of pharmaceutical companies on prescribing practices often distorts the nature of care and is contributing to irrational care. It promotes prescriptions which are not backed by the standard guidelines given in textbooks.

3. There is a lot of dissatisfaction in many quarters concerning 'donation'-charging private medical colleges, which produce doctors who have paid enormous amounts of money, running into millions of rupees, to obtain their degrees. The large numbers of such doctors entering the medical field with the primary objective of 'recovering' their investment fuels and significantly promotes the gross commercialization of medical services.

4. Some doctors are of the firm opinion that generic medicines should be prescribed in preference to branded medicines.

(For example, the basic ingredient in 'Crocin' and 'Calpol' branded tablets is paracetamol.) Patients should be able to access cheap yet good quality medicines under their generic name.

5. There is a definite and urgent need for effective regulation of the private medical sector.

6. As part of regulating the health care sector, it is possible to ensure standard treatment guidelines. Such provisions need to be introduced even though some doctors argue that it is impossible to introduce standard treatment guidelines. The doctors we interviewed have contested this assertion. Our doctors are clearly telling us that not only is it possible to bring in standard treatment guidelines, but it is essential to do so.

7. Rates for different types of hospitals and services, and for various categories of cities/towns, can be standardized and a range can be defined, at least for beds in the general ward, semi-private and private wards. Many of our doctors support the creation of a practical range list of standard rates.

8. Official medical councils, which are supposed to regulate the private medical sector, have so far largely failed to do so. These bodies have themselves become part of the system. We need to change the nature of these organizations and make them socially responsive.

9. There is need for change in social attitudes as well. Health care is a social right; it is not a mere commodity to be sold and purchased. In the realm of health care, 'more' is not necessarily 'better' and 'most expensive' is not necessarily 'best'. In many situations, simple measures may be preferable to excessive interventions. There is need for social attitudes to move away from 'medical consumerism' and 'doctor-shopping'. People need to be aware of the limits and strengths of various systems of healing and their distinctive modes of treatment. There is a need for widespread sensitization on all these issues.

It would not be wrong to say that these points, which our doctors largely agree upon, can be a starting point for a roadmap for reform in the private medical sector in India.

Building upon these suggestions, in this second part of the book, we will discuss what can be done to address the current situation and to promote change, concerning the private medical sector. In the coming pages, we will outline possible strategies at two levels:

1. At Individual Level

- Knowing about patients' rights, so that basic entitlements can be asked for in private hospitals (Chapter 8)
- Understanding how to choose a rational, ethical doctor (Chapter 9)

2. At Social and Policy Level

- Working for effective, socially responsive regulation of the private medical sector (Chapter 10)
- Moving towards a system of Universal Health Care (Chapter 11)
- Contributing to collective forums, broad movements to achieve policy changes, as well as reshaping social attitudes concerning health (Chapter 12)

No doubt we are dealing with a complicated case—a long-standing malady—hence the cure may also be somewhat complex, and might take some time. But there can be no disagreement that the treatment must be started in real earnest now. Since this is a problem of social dimensions, not only for the medical profession, but also affecting various sections of society—citizens' groups, social organizations, policymakers, and ordinary people—we will need to put in substantial energies and efforts to tackle the malaise that besets the private medical sector in India today.

Chapter 8

What Rights Do I Have as a Patient in a Private Hospital?

Most of us do not think in terms of 'rights' when we ourselves, or someone close to us, is admitted into a private hospital. Perhaps we have been conditioned to think of seeking care in a private hospital as a purely commercial transaction. However, it is important to know that we have definite entitlements even in the context of private doctors and hospitals, even though today in India these rights need further strengthening in a legal framework.

Firstly, we may keep in mind that we have rights as consumers—whether we are buying a packet of milk, a pair of shoes or a car. Health care services are covered by the Consumer Protection Act (CPA), and in case of medical negligence, claims for compensation can be made in a consumer redressal forum. However, this mechanism is limited to cases of medical negligence, and it does not take into account the wider spectrum of health care rights. We will touch upon the complexities of CPA in the context of health care later in this chapter, but we should keep in mind that this is one form of protection of our rights as consumers in private hospitals.

Secondly, health care is not just like any other commodity, but is a special kind of service that deals with life and death situations. There is a special kind of relationship between doctors and patients, which is characterized by major imbalances of power and knowledge. Doctors take or guide many decisions on behalf of patients, and they exercise certain types of power over the recipients of their services, which is unique among various professions. Society has also historically awarded certain status and privileges to medical professionals, given their special role. Considering this entire context, health care needs to be regulated by a framework of ethics and protective provisions unlike most other services. We do have certain specific rights in the case of health care providers, including private providers, even though these need to be more clearly defined and legally operationalized in the Indian context.

There are several frameworks and justifications that support such entitlements for patients in the context of health care. The Medical Council of India, which is supposed to regulate the conduct of doctors in India, has a 'Code of Medical Ethics Regulations'.[1] This code specifies the ethical guidelines to be observed by doctors during their dealings with patients, with each other, with the general public, and with the pharmaceutical industry. Unfortunately, in practice this important code seems to be a kind of well-kept secret, since it has hardly ever been publicized, and the key provisions from the viewpoint of patients (which we will describe below) are unknown to most people. This code is hardly given any importance in the medical curriculum, with the consequence that it is rarely given much importance even by doctors themselves.

Further, the Supreme Court of India has made certain important judgements and has issued orders in specific cases that cover patients' rights. In addition, Chhattisgarh is one Indian state which legally protects patients' rights through its Clinical Establishments Act (which covers all health care establishments including private hospitals and nursing homes); in fact there is a strong case that the national Clinical Establishments Act and similar acts in various states of India should include similar provisions to protect patients' rights. India is also a signatory to various international human rights covenants, which specify the need to protect the rights of patients in all kinds of health care institutions, including private hospitals.

Taking into account this entire context, we can propose a Charter of Patients' Rights, which draws upon various existing provisions in the Indian context. The rights outlined below are significantly based on the 'Charter of Patients' Rights and Responsibilities' which was drafted through discussion and consensus among patients' rights groups and representatives of private doctors in Pune[2] in 2006.

1. RIGHT TO EMERGENCY MEDICAL CARE

As per Supreme Court directives, all doctors, both in the government and in the private sector, are duty-bound to provide basic Emergency Medical Care, and injured persons have a right to get Emergency Medical Care.[3] Inability to pay on behalf of the patient cannot be a basis for denying emergency treatment.[4] The MCI Code of Ethics also specifies that doctors should not neglect or avoid treating patients during emergencies.[5] Basic emergency treatment would consist of some essential measures like removing any blockages in the respiratory passage, checking blood loss, giving intravenous fluids etc., and preparation for referral to another appropriate hospital if required. Only after providing this basic emergency care, hospitals should demand fees or can start informing the police. The National Consumer Disputes Redressal Commission has given a clear opinion on this, in the case of Sumanta Mukherjee.

> **The Sad Case of Sumanta Mukherjee—**
> **and the Lesson for Hospitals Concerning Emergency**
> **Medical Care**
>
> On 14 January, 2001, Sumanta Mukherjee, an electrical engineering student, aged twenty, was going to attend his tuition class on a motorcycle and was knocked down from behind by a bus of the Calcutta Tram Company. Sumanta, who was conscious after the accident, was taken to a private

hospital, which was around 1 km from the accident site, by a crowd of people that had gathered there after the accident.

Sumanta was insured under Mediclaim policy for Rs 65,000, and at the time of reaching the Hospital, he was conscious and showed his Mediclaim certificate, which he was carrying in his wallet, to the attending doctor and hospital staff. He promised them that the charges for the treatment would be paid and that they should start the treatment. The hospital started the treatment in its Emergency Room by giving oxygen and some emergency medicines; however, after starting the treatment they began to insist upon immediate payment of Rs 15,000, and threatened to discontinue treatment if it was not immediately deposited. Various persons present in the group accompanying Sumanta requested the hospital staff to continue treating him, and assured them that the payment would be made as soon as they were able to get in touch with Sumanta's parents. The crowd present there also offered to pay Rs 2000 and to handover Sumanta's motorcycle to the hospital, while the Mediclaim certificate was also showed again.

The hospital, however, remained adamant about the immediate deposit of Rs 15,000 and showing gross deficiency in service in utter violation of medical ethics, they discontinued the treatment. Persons from the crowd present were then forced to take Sumanta to the National Calcutta Medical College and Hospital, which is about 7 to 8 km from the private hospital. Sumanta died on the way and was declared dead at said hospital.

Sumanta's father lodged a complaint with the National Consumer Disputes Redressal Commission, which in its order opined that 'deficiency in service on the part of the respondents (hospital and staff) is apparent' and ordered them to pay compensation of Rs 10 lakh to Sumanta's family. The Consumer Disputes Redressal Commission noted in its order, while recommending compensation, that:

> 'This may serve the purpose of bringing about a qualitative change in the attitude of the hospitals of providing service to the human beings as human beings. Human touch is necessary; that is their code of conduct; that is their duty and that is what is required to be implemented. In emergency or critical cases let them discharge their duty/social obligation of rendering service without waiting for fees or for consent.'

The right to emergency medical care becomes especially important in case of accidents and major injuries, where prompt initiation of emergency treatment may make the difference between life and death. In such situations, if a hospital insists on advance payment before starting treatment, it is both unethical and contrary to law. At the same time, while not diluting the basic right, it may be kept in mind that smaller nursing homes or specialized clinics may not have the means to provide certain kinds of emergency care beyond the most basic measures. It has also been argued that a public fund should be set up to ensure free emergency treatment to poor patients, who may be unable to pay the charges, so that individual hospitals may not have to regularly subsidize such free care to poor patients from their own resources.

2. Right to Information, Including Information about Rates of Services

All patients should be given adequate, relevant information about the nature, severity and likely outcome of their present illness; provisional diagnosis or confirmed diagnosis; professional charges of the doctor;[6] relevant information about the proposed care; the expected results, risks and advantages of various alternative procedures; and the treatment options available. However, it should be noted that sometimes a precise diagnosis may not be initially possible, and there are no set standards about exactly how much information is to be given. Hence, what minimum information is to be provided has to be more clearly defined, based on practical experience.

**Fast Surgeon, Slow with Giving Information—
Testimony by a Doctor about His Senior
(Incident recounted by a doctor to one of the authors)**

I remember even today what I experienced in my residency in a large hospital in Mumbai. Our surgeon boss always boasted that he was the fastest surgeon in the world. He was very skilful and did miracles of performing surgeries at breathtaking speed. One day, he started to remove a stone from a patient's kidney and set a target of ten minutes—from opening the skin to sewing up the skin. But luck was not with him on that day; due to sheer hurry he accidentally cut the main artery to the kidney. Because of this mistake, he had to remove the entire kidney, rather than only removing the stone.

Afterwards he explained dramatically to the relatives about how the kidney had been damaged by the stone, and hence how fortunate the patient was to have been managed by himself—a skilful surgeon. The relatives thanked him profusely, but I was amazed by how rank negligence was hidden under false information. The casualty was not just the patient's kidney, but also his right to information!

Doctors may take the help of informative booklets written in simple language and comprehensible to patients, or any educational material, or may take the help of assistant doctors or nurses to provide relevant information to the patient. Any queries beyond what can be answered by assistants should be addressed by the concerned main doctor. Patients or persons authorized by the patient should be informed about the likely cost of the treatment in advance. The patient and family should be informed about the financial implications, when there is a change in the patient's condition or line of treatment.

For the benefit of patients, rates charged for each type of service provided and facilities available, should be displayed at a conspicuous place in the hospital, in the local language as well as in English.[7] It is further highly desirable that the hospital provide a brochure of standard rates to the admitted patient/caregivers. This should include rates for major services relevant to the patient such as rates for a normal and caesarean delivery, for routine tests (like routine blood, urine, X-ray, sonography examination), specialist's fee for each visit etc. This will help the patient to figure out the likely expenditure during the course of hospitalization. Hospitals should clearly inform and display that such a rate card is available to all patients.

On request, the hospital should provide written expenditure estimation to patients according to his or her illness and planned treatment. The patient or person authorized by the patient should be informed about the financial implications, when there is a change in the patient's condition or treatment setting.

3. RIGHT TO MEDICAL REPORTS AND RECORDS

This is an extension of the Right to Information. The patient or a person authorized by the patient has a right to have access to his or her indoor case paper's photocopy (during period of admission, preferably within 24 hours, and after discharge, within 72 hours) after paying the appropriate fees for photocopying.[8]

The patient has a right to his or her medical record and no hospital, public or private, can deny a patient their records and reports,[9] including reports of diagnostic tests, opinions expressed by doctors or specialists, reason for admission in hospital etc.

How a Publisher Was Denied His Wife's Critical Sonography Report
(Personal experience recounted to one of the authors)

My wife was seven months pregnant, and she was registered with a reputed gynaecologist in Pune. One evening, she had mild pain in her abdomen, mostly gas trouble. We did not want to take any chances and hence visited the gynaecologist, who ordered a sonography. When he read the report, he advised us to get admitted immediately, for applying a stitch on the cervix (mouth of the uterus) on an emergency basis. He warned that if we did not do so, he could not guarantee the safety of the baby, and there was risk of miscarriage.

Being a publisher, I called one of our contributing authors who is a gynaecologist as well (Dr Arun Gadre). He listened to the story and assured me that given the history, there was probably no need to put a stitch. However, he advised me to bring the sonography report. When I demanded one from the hospital, the treating gynaecologist became angry; he simply declared that his hospital's policy is not to give any reports to the patient. I was furious. Then my wife and I left this hospital and visited another gynaecologist, suggested by my author friend. The second gynaecologist laughed when she heard the history; she examined my wife and declared that even sonography was not required, and there was definitely no need to put a stitch. Just to alleviate our anxiety she ordered a sonography, whose report came out to be perfectly normal. My wife subsequently had a normal, full term pregnancy and delivery, and we now have a lovely baby!

How can doctors deny giving the patient their reports? When we have paid for the investigation, performed on our own body, how could they refuse to give reports which rightfully belong to us?

At the time of discharge, the patient should get a discharge card, which should contain: the condition of the patient at the time of admission, important clinical findings, summarized results of laboratory tests, diagnosis and treatment during hospitalization, the condition of the patient at discharge, date of follow-up visit if required, and medicines and precautions to be taken after discharge. Clear instructions should be given in cases where certain medicines should not be stopped without a doctor's consultation (e.g., medicines for high blood pressure, diabetes etc.) and instructions should be given regarding possible emergency situations. This follow-up advice should be written in a language and manner which can be easily understood by a common person.

In case of death of a patient, the death summary should be provided to the deceased's relatives. It should include all important medical points, ranging from the condition of the patient at the time of admission, to the cause of death.[10]

4. RIGHT TO SEEK SECOND OPINION

In our country, patients are often hesitant to seek a second opinion, even if they have doubts concerning the diagnosis or line of treatment being suggested by a doctor. However, there is no basis to deny any patient the right to seek a second opinion, with due information about this being given to the primary treating doctor. Broadly there is consensus among experts that patients have a right to seek a second opinion.[11] All copies of medical and diagnostic reports should be made available to the patient or authorized caregiver, to facilitate a second opinion. No rationally practising, ethical doctor should feel offended in case a patient seeks a second opinion; in fact doctors should welcome an additional expert opinion being given, which may help to clarify the diagnosis or may refine the line of treatment.

Seeking a second opinion may be especially important when the diagnosis is unclear, when the suspected condition is life-threatening, or when a major procedure or operation is being considered. Besides contacting individual doctors, in India now some online second opinion services are also available, which offer such expert opinion for a fee.

5. RIGHT TO CONFIDENTIALITY AND PRIVACY DURING TREATMENT

Patients reveal many aspects of their personal lives to their doctors, since such information may be essential to reach a diagnosis, or the personal habits and lifestyle of the patient may have a bearing on the treatment process. This may include drinking and smoking habits, sexual histories and preferences, and details of marital and family life. Patients often need to bare their bodies and even their minds to doctors, sharing sensitive information, which might not be normally revealed to others. Given this context, patients have a right to privacy, and doctors have a duty to hold such information in strict confidentiality, unless it is essential in specific circumstances, to communicate such information to protect others.[12]

Denial of Privacy and Confidentiality, Combined with Discrimination
(Recounted by one of the authors)

I remember that when the HIV epidemic was at its peak, I got a call from a fellow doctor at 2 a.m. She narrated how she had driven out an HIV positive patient with labour pains from her hospital, and gave me a warning that the patient might be coming to my hospital. She felt she was doing her 'duty' to save a fellow doctor from getting exposed to an HIV positive patient! I did not heed her advice, since I never refused HIV positive patients. But I wondered how a doctor could drive away a patient in labour just because she is HIV positive? And what about the confidentiality of that patient? The HIV report that this doctor shared with me was not a routine transfer of information between two doctors in the best interests of the patient, rather it was a breach of privacy and confidentiality, the fundamental rights of any patient.

6. Right to Informed Consent, Before Undergoing a Potentially Hazardous Test or Operation

A doctor may recommend to a particular patient that he or she needs to undergo an invasive test (such as an angiography) or an operation or major procedure, which carries certain risks. In such cases, it is obligatory for the doctor to explain to the patient and caregivers the main risks that are involved in the procedure, and after giving this information, the doctor may proceed only if consent has been giving in writing by the patient/caregiver. As far as possible (except in emergencies), adequate time should be given to the patient/caregivers to decide, after understanding the risks, whether they want to proceed with the test/operation or not. This requirement is clearly specified in the MCI Code of Ethics.[13]

In practice, often such consent is obtained in a perfunctory manner. Maybe just minutes before the operation, the patient or relative may be asked to quickly sign a consent form, without properly explaining the risks, and without giving the patient and caregivers adequate time to make an informed decision. Keeping such possibilities in mind, if the patient or caregivers know that some invasive test or operation is likely to be recommended, they should tell the doctor to inform them about the risks and implications in advance, and should not be pushed into undergoing any procedure, without first having been explained the risks and possible outcomes.

7. Right to Choice of Medical Store or Diagnostic Centre

It is a common experience for the relatives and friends of a patient admitted in a hospital to be told 'buy these medicines, but only from the pharmacy in our hospital', or 'get this test done, but only from so-and-so laboratory'. One may wonder why in a so-called 'free market' scenario, where the 'consumer is king', such irrational and binding conditions are specified by certain hospitals, and the reality becomes, 'consumer is slave'. Not infrequently, the same medicine bought from the hospital pharmacy may be found to be much more expensive than the same medicine, or another brand of the same medicine made by a standard company, if bought elsewhere. The reason being that many hospitals earn significant income by renting out space to a medical store, and then allow the store to charge for medicines liberally from the patient. However, forcing patients to buy medicines from a particular store is not only unethical, it has also been ruled by consumer disputes redressal commissions to be a violation of the consumers' rights .

Consumer Launches a Legal Battle for the Right to Choose Source of Medicine

In January 2009, Shri Ganesh Kelkar had his grandson admitted in a leading private hospital in Pune for treatment of a serious disease. Since the cost of medicine provided by the hospital was very high, amounting to about Rs 1,50,000 for fifteen injections, he consulted a family member who was a doctor to explore any way of getting this medicine at a lower cost. The doctor from the patient's family assured him that the same medicine could be obtained from another source at 60 per cent of the mentioned MRP. Shri Kelkar approached the hospital, asking them if they would allow the family to buy the same medicine from another source. The hospital management flatly refused, and stated that they would have to buy this expensive medicine (at much higher rate) from the hospital's pharmacy at MRP, otherwise he should get the child discharged. Not having much choice, the family got the child treated while accessing the expensive medicine provided by the hospital. Although the hospital later gave an 8 per cent discount, still the Kelkar family had to shell out around Rs 50,000 extra because they were not allowed to buy the same brand at 40 per cent of discount from another source in the market.

After the child was treated and discharged, Shri Kelkar filed a case in the District Consumer Redressal Forum in December 2009, complaining that his rights as a consumer had been violated. Shri Kelkar asked the hospital to pay to make up the financial loss of Rs 50,000 and Rs 3000 towards the legal costs, but asked that the hospital pay a token compensation of only one rupee for the harassment caused! It was clear that he was not hankering after the money, but rather wanted to teach a lesson to the hospital, which had denied his basic right as a consumer. In its judgement in October 2012, the District Consumer Forum upheld Kelkar's argument, and ruled that the hospital had indulged in unfair trade practice. But strangely enough, the Forum declined the demand for payment of Rs 50,000 on the grounds that the hospital had not charged above the MRP. The hospital next appealed against this order in the State Consumer Forum at Mumbai. This appeal is now being fought on technical grounds of procedures, and the final judgement is yet to come, six years after the case was launched. Mr Kelkar's struggle to seek redressal for denial of a basic and justified consumer right continues!

There is a similar, recent case of a leading hospital in Jaipur, associated with a national corporate hospital chain. A particular woman patient had a serious condition for which the hospital prescribed certain expensive injections. Initially the cost of each injection was cited as Rs 9000. However, at the time of discharge, the patient was billed at the rate of Rs 18,990 per injection for a total of twenty-five injections, supplied from the hospital pharmacy.

The husband of the patient had requested the hospital authorities that the concerned injection was available at 30–40 per cent discount in other medical shops in the market, and he appealed to the hospital to be permitted to purchase the injections from outside. But this request was rejected and he was forced to purchase the injections from the hospital itself.

The patient's husband later filed a complaint in the District Consumer Forum, claiming that excessive money had been charged by the hospital; this forum ruled in the patient's favour. The hospital appealed against this decision and went to the State Consumer Commission, which also ruled in the patient's favour. Finally the issue was raised in the National Consumer Disputes Redressal Commission, which stated that:[14]

'We are of the opinion that the hospital authorities exercised undue influence and compelled the Complainants to pay an excess price. This amounts to unfair trade practice. The right of the Complainant/patient cannot be curtailed, by preventing the Complainants to exercise their option to purchase the medicines or injections from the market.'

Keeping in view various factors, the National Commission ordered the hospital to pay 50 per cent of the excess amount charged by them, to the patient's family. However, the overall legal situation is clear—no hospital can force a patient or their family to buy specified medicines only from their own hospital pharmacy; they are free to purchase the same medicine from any other source.

It may also be kept in mind that the Medical Council of India Code of Ethics for doctors specifies that all doctors should as far as possible prescribe medicines by generic names,[15] that is the scientific name which is independent of particular brand names. This naturally implies that the patient would be free to choose any standard brand of the medicine, from any store of choice. Hence, whenever faced with the condition 'buy the medicines only from our hospital store', while we might sometimes consider the convenience of buying from the same hospital, if we are aware of significant cost differences, then we should feel free to purchase the same standard medicine from any store or source of our choice.

8. Right to Comprehensive Protection, When the Patient Is Being Involved in a Clinical Trial

Nowadays it is not uncommon for patients to be enrolled in trials of new medicines, especially in case of certain serious illnesses where new, experimental treatments are being tested. India is a 'destination of choice' for multinational drug companies, which find it easier and cheaper to test a new drug in India compared to developed countries, due to much less stringent regulations and lower operational costs here. However, the downside of this situation is that the rights of patients involved in the testing of new drugs may be seriously violated. Several studies have documented serious violations of patients' rights during clinical trials in India[16,17,18]; and a major campaign and Supreme Court case has been launched by the civil society group 'Swasthya Adhikar Manch'[19] to ensure justice to the survivors and families of patients who have suffered from unethical practices during clinical trials in India. The Indian Council of Medical Research (ICMR) has clearly laid down certain basic ethical guidelines that must be followed during any trial of an experimental medicine or intervention.[20] This is a major issue of concern that has been dealt with in detail by various official bodies and civil society organizations; here we will just summarize some of the rights of patients that must be protected if they are enrolled in any clinical trials, which are often carried out in the context of private hospitals (this section is substantially based on the above mentioned ICMR guidelines):

a. **Participation must be based on consent, given after provision of complete information**
   Several studies and interviews of participants in clinical trials in India have shown that persons enrolled in such trials are often not given proper information about the trial, and that their consent was obtained without providing such basic information. The medical researcher must obtain informed consent of the participant, based on providing full information about the nature and purpose of the study,

various details including possible risks and discomforts which should be properly described, availability of medical treatment for any injuries or adverse effects related to the trial, information about any alternative treatments if available, and full contact details of the main researchers.

It should also be clearly communicated that free treatment would be made available by the researchers for any research-related adverse effects, and that participants would be eligible for compensation for any disability or death resulting from such injury. The fact that any individual or family has the freedom to participate and to withdraw from research at any time, without any loss of benefits, should also be clearly mentioned. The patient should be given a copy of the signed informed consent form, which provides him or her with a record containing basic information about the trial, and also becomes documentary evidence to prove their participation in the trial. The patient should also be informed in writing about the name of the drug that is undergoing trial, along with dates, dose and duration of administration.

b. **Compensation for injury or disability, entitlement to treatment for side effects**

Research participants who suffer physical injury as a result of their participation in a trial are entitled to financial or other assistance, to compensate them for any impairment or disability. In the case of death, their dependents have the right to compensation.

For participants who experience any adverse reactions to a vaccine or drug under trial, the best possible nationally available care must be made available free of cost, and as long as required. The expenses on treatment and financial compensation for any trial-related injury or death of the clinical trial participant must be borne by the sponsor of the trial.

c. **Insurance coverage and compensation for participation**

In many clinical trials, participants may be entitled to payment for the time they spend and the discomfort they experience, and they should be reimbursed for any expenses that they have to make related to their participation in research, which may include daily wages and travel expenses. Guidelines require that trial participants must be given proper insurance coverage, or should have an adequate compensation scheme related to the trial.

d. Access to benefits after the trial has been completed

The liability of the researchers to participants does not end with the trial. The World Medical Assembly (WMA)[21] states that after the trial, participants should be assured of access to the best treatment methods that may have been proven by the study. Participants, who still need an intervention that may have been identified as beneficial in the trial, should be provided the same. If the medicine that was being tried out is subsequently found to be effective, the trial participants are entitled to receive that drug either free of cost or at a subsidized rate.

Victim of an Unethical Clinical Trial

Mr Shrikrishna Gehlod from Indore had a chronic lung problem, and had difficulty breathing. In January 2009, he was admitted into a large government hospital in Indore, where he was asked to sign some papers, while the doctors told him they would treat him with some drugs imported from America. He was not informed at any stage that he was being enrolled in a trial for an experimental drug. He was periodically admitted for 15–20 days at a time on four occasions over a year, and each time the experimental drug was administered to him through an inhaler. Following this treatment, Mr Gehlod's breathing problems significantly increased, his health started deteriorating, and he became unable to carry out his normal work. No insurance was provided, nor was any care given to him following the trial. After realizing that he had been

unknowingly enrolled in a clinical trial which had worsened
his health, he complained to the National Human Rights
Commission in 2011 and asked for compensation for damage
to his health, along with an inquiry into the entire process of
this unethical trial. Mr Gehlod's health continued to worsen
and he breathed his last in January 2012. The family has been
asking for documents and details of this trial conducted by
the multinational drug company, but the medical investigators
have not even bothered to respond to the queries.

Source: Swasthya Adhikar Manch

9. Right to Take Discharge of Patient, or Receive Body of Deceased from Hospital, Regardless of Payment of Complete Hospital Bill

It is becoming a rather common practice among certain hospitals to
refuse to release a patient until the complete hospital bills have been
paid, thus detaining the patient. Perhaps even worse are incidents
of certain hospitals refusing to handover the dead body of a patient,
until the complete bill has been paid. The Bombay High Court has
noted that the practice of hospitals detaining patients is contrary
to law, and amounts to 'illegal detention'[22] (see box). Similar legal
opinions have been expressed by courts, censuring hospitals which
have not given dead bodies of patients to relatives on grounds that
the complete bill was not paid.

Patient Held Hostage over Payment of Disputed Bill, High Court Terms It 'Illegal Detention'[23,24]

Following a head injury in March 2014, a young man was
admitted and operated upon in a leading private hospital in

Mumbai. The family paid Rs 2.76 lakh to the hospital for the treatment. The brother of the patient felt that the patient's condition was not improving as expected, and decided to shift him elsewhere. But the hospital insisted on additional payment of a large amount, which was disputed by the brother, and the hospital allegedly refused to release the patient until the disputed bills were paid.

The brother of the patient approached the Bombay High Court, where judges of the division bench denounced as 'inhuman' the practice of certain hospitals detaining patients until their medical bills were paid. The Court also observed that nowadays 'doctors have forgotten their duty' and that this was no less than 'illegal detention' by the hospital. The government pleader in the case stated that there is no law that provides hospitals the right to detain patients for non-payment of dues, or to keep the body of a dead patient for such a reason. The patient in this case was finally discharged without the family paying the additional disputed amount, and the hospital later denied that they had detained the patient.

Naturally, the hospital should inform the patient and family about the total expected costs of treatment in advance, and should practise daily billing with details to prevent such disputes about billing around the time of discharge. However, in case of any disputes over billing, detaining a patient or refusing to handover the dead body of a deceased patient must be treated as an unethical and illegal practice.

We have outlined above some of the rights to protect patients in the context of hospitals, including private hospitals. The basis for these rights, as pointed out, is the Code of Medical Ethics that governs doctors, as well as certain judgements of courts and consumer redressal forums. Let us now briefly see how these rights can be claimed.

How Can We Claim Patients' Rights?

In case, as a patient or caregiver, we perceive that any of these rights is being violated, then wherever feasible, we should gather the full details of the case and consult a local consumer organization or organization working on health rights. Based on such advice, along with concrete evidence of violation of rights, the patient or caregiver should first of all enter into a dialogue with the hospital management and concerned doctor, to ensure that the violation is corrected or prevented. Here it is useful to keep in mind that the involved doctor and the hospital management are often not identical, and some doctors may be more sympathetic and sensitive to ethical concerns raised by the patient, compared to commercial hospital managements. During such a dialogue, while giving sound justification, attempts should be made to convince the doctor and hospital to fulfil the rights of the patient and to stop/prevent any perceived violation.

If this initial step does not succeed, then depending on the nature of the violation, there are a few forms of recourse presently available. In case one experiences that a doctor has violated the Code of Medical Ethics, the patient or caregiver can make a complaint to the State Medical Council.

Medical Councils—
Bodies Supposed to Ensure Ethical Conduct by Doctors[25]

Medical Councils are legal bodies, which are supposed to govern the medical profession. Councils cannot give compensation to a complainant, and the only punishment the councils can hand out to a doctor is cancellation of the registration of a doctor, on a temporary or permanent basis. The complaint needs to be submitted to the registrar of the Council, in a prescribed format. The executive committee of the state council holds a preliminary hearing to determine whether the complaint should be further dealt with. At this preliminary meeting, only the person making the complaint and the doctor against whom the complaint is filed, are allowed to present their versions; lawyers are not allowed to be present. If the executive committee finds some validity in the complaint, then the full medical council hears the case. However, it may be kept in mind that the full medical council generally meets only twice in a year, and many state councils are presently understaffed. In this situation, complaints are often not resolved in a timely manner. Further, as can be imagined, since the preliminary hearing involves only doctors from the executive committee of the council, and the complainant is generally a layperson, this is heavily tilted against the person making the complaint, because of vast differences in level of medical knowledge. Due to this entire situation, so far medical councils in India have not been particularly effective in resolving the complaints of ordinary patients.

Medical Negligence and Consumer Protection Act

Another major kind of violation that patients might suffer from is medical negligence. This is a specialized subject on which several books and articles have been written,[26,27,28] which can be consulted for those interested in detailed information. Hence we are not dealing with medical negligence in depth in this chapter; rather a very brief overview of the related consumer protection mechanism is given here.

Any doctor owes to his or her patient a certain basic standard of care. If this care has not been properly delivered, leading to damage to the patient, then this is considered to be an instance of medical negligence. In India, medical services are covered by the Consumer Protection Act (CPA), hence if there is a perceived case of medical negligence, a patient or family member can approach the relevant consumer redressal forum. The main plea that is often made in such forums is the demand for compensation, due to negligence on behalf of the doctor or care provider. Consumer redressal forums and commissions, to hear such cases, have been set up at district, state and national levels in India. Complaints can be filed in the District Forum if the compensation claimed is less than Rs 20 lakh, at the State Commission if the compensation claimed is within Rs 1 crore, or at the National Commission if the compensation exceeds Rs 1 crore.

However, it may be kept in mind that the complaint of negligence against a doctor needs generally to be accompanied by an expert opinion from another doctor of the concerned specialization, stating that the complaint appears valid on first examination, and deserves further investigation. Without such a certificate, a complaint of medical negligence is not likely to be admitted. Further, all relevant medical records and reports would also need to be submitted along with the complaint.

In medical negligence cases, the patient has to establish his or her case against the doctor, rather than the doctor having to prove his or her innocence; negligence has to be established and cannot be presumed. While there are certain cases in India where patients have managed to obtain substantial compensation amounts, in the large majority of cases filed, it has been difficult to prove clearly that negligence has taken place. Moreover, the CPA mechanism tends to create an adversarial situation between the patient and doctor in a buyer–seller type of framework, and is suitable only for dealing with cases of serious negligence. It is not a comprehensive mechanism to deal with the wider spectrum of patients' rights issues, and is not primarily a preventive mechanism. Hence, while certain patients who have suffered serious negligence in the form of grossly substandard care may adopt the CPA route, it should be emphasized that there is also definitely need for broader and more wide-ranging mechanisms to protect and promote patients' rights.

Here, it should also be noted that technically, patients can also file a case in a civil court, in case of a complaint against a hospital, claiming damages. However, this is not likely to be very effective, since it may easily take more than a decade for any kind of decision to be taken. Currently over 30 million cases are pending in numerous courts across India. At the current rate, analysts say that it could take anywhere between 350 to 400 years to sort out the entire legal backlog! Given this general background of our legal system, there is not much chance that going to the civil court to complain against medical negligence would provide justice to patients. It is no wonder that civil courts have played a negligible role in regulating the private medical sector.

Given This Situation, How Can We Qualitatively Strengthen Implementation of Patients' Rights?

Of course, wherever required and appropriate, patients and their caregivers should consider using the redressal mechanisms mentioned above. However, given the current limitations of medical councils, and the limited focus of the Consumer Protection Act, today in India there is need for a comprehensive mechanism that would enable patients to claim their rights, which would provide patient-friendly redressal, and would prevent violations in a much more effective manner. These mechanisms should be applicable to hospitals and other health care establishments and not just doctors, which happens to be the case with the current Code of Medical Ethics. Also, issues like standards of care, ensuring availability of necessary infrastructure and equipment, and following of appropriate processes while treating patients should be covered by such a mechanism. This is possible if patients' rights are covered in Clinical Establishment Acts as a required process standard to be ensured by all hospitals. We discuss this in Chapter 10.

Chapter 9

How Can I Recognize a Rational, Ethical Doctor?

In the previous chapter, we had a look at the basic rights of patients which are mandatory for any doctor or hospital to observe. These are the bare minimum norms of conduct that we are entitled to expect from any health care provider. But obviously our expectations do not stop at this minimum level! We would always prefer a doctor who would give us rational, good quality care in an ethical and humane manner. Yet from the first part of this book—and our own experience as health care consumers—we know that not all doctors today are equally rational and ethical in their practice. At the same time, the difference between a rational, ethical doctor and one who is not so, can be the crucial difference between good health outcomes and bad health outcomes, and sometimes even between life and death. Given the fact that we may have the chance to interact with any doctor on only a few occasions, and may have limited choices, it is important to know how to recognize whether a doctor is rational and ethical overall, or not. As doctors who have practised ourselves, and have interacted with many other doctors, we give a few clues about how to spot a good doctor, not just based on looking at technical qualifications, but based on the doctor's mode of interacting with patients.

A rational, ethical doctor,
- Does not mind being asked questions by the patient
- Gives sufficient information, enabling the patient/caregivers to understand the course of illness and treatment
- Gives the patient various options whenever possible, and discusses pros and cons, enabling the patient and caregivers to take an appropriate decision
- Explains to the patient the justification for any major investigations and invasive procedures being ordered

The most important asymmetry between a doctor and patient is the asymmetry of knowledge. The doctor generally knows much more about what is going on in the patient's body, what needs to be done about the same, and what is the likely outcome, than what most patients will ever know. Such asymmetry of knowledge is rather inevitable, given the vast and complex nature of modern medical science. However, given this context, the doctor has a duty to share a small portion of his or her vast pool of knowledge with the patient—at the very least by carefully answering the questions and doubts of the patient and caregivers; and by allowing the patient and caregivers the autonomy of choosing among appropriate treatment options, wherever applicable. Hence when we choose a doctor, one of the most important considerations we may keep in mind besides technical skills, is the doctor's willingness to talk, explain and offer reasonable options.

One case from Dr Arun Gadre's experience is quite illustrative of the importance of these attributes in a doctor.

A ninety-year-old man was admitted at midnight into a reputed nursing home, with heart failure and severe breathlessness. The relatives were anxious, since even though they knew that age was catching up with Grandpa, his present suffering was unbearable. The physician came and prescribed something; he was not ready to entertain any questions. His blunt response was: 'What can we do for a person at the age of ninety with such severe heart failure?' When the patient's son tried to inquire about how to lessen the old man's suffering, the rude answer came, 'Do not argue with me, I have no time to answer silly questions.'

Grandpa was shifted to another hospital, because his grandson was a surgeon, who reached home from another city in a timely manner, and intervened in the management. Now another physician was consulted, who patiently answered all the questions and elaborated upon the nearly hopeless long-term prognosis for the elderly man, but agreed to perform a small procedure to remove the liquid that had collected around his lungs, and thus to relieve him of his severe suffering due to breathlessness. The simple process of dialogue between the patient's caregivers and the doctor made a huge difference.

The message is simple—whenever there is a choice between two doctors with similar years of experience and qualifications, opt for the doctor who is willing to talk with you and explain things. The practice of medicine is not just about good technical skills, to a great extent it is also about good communication. The very word 'doctor' is derived from the Latin word for 'teacher'. Unfortunately, lured by the desire for making more money, and by taking on more and more patients but talking less and less with them, some doctors seem to have forgotten the original meaning of their designation 'Dr', which almost becomes their second name. Many of the disputes in hospitals, and much of the dissatisfaction among patients related to health care today, stem from inadequate communication by providers, and patients not being given sufficient information.

In brief, whenever we are in the role of a patient or caregiver, we should try to choose providers who are willing and able to communicate—every patient deserves to be talked to decently, and given an explanation about their illness and the treatment that they are undergoing.

A rational, ethical doctor does not create fear or panic, but gives timely and balanced information.

It has been said that if you can make a person sufficiently fearful, you can get him to do almost anything. And there is perhaps nothing that induces as much fear as the apprehension of physical suffering or loss of life. In this context, when a patient approaches a doctor, there is a valid expectation that while the severity of the problem should not be underplayed, the patient should not be driven into panic and rushed into taking a major decision like undergoing an operation (except of course in the case of genuine emergencies). Unfortunately nowadays instances of such 'panic-inducing medical advice' are becoming rather common. We have not infrequently come across situations where immediately after an angiography, the cardiologist has told the patient that 'angioplasty must be done immediately, within a few hours'—and the patient has been rushed into undergoing an invasive procedure, even though the option of waiting and taking a balanced decision might have proved to be more appropriate. The following experience illustrates this kind of problem quite well.

Dr Arun Gadre has a friend whose daughter is an athlete, who loves to exercise. One day her knee got unlocked and she fell down suddenly while just standing! Concerned about the fall, my friend took her to an orthopaedic surgeon, and the MRI confirmed that she had torn her knee ligaments while exercising. The surgeon advised laparoscopic surgery of the knee joint. When asked about the consequences if the surgery was avoided, he plainly threatened that her knee joint would get ruined, she would get severe arthritis, and in the end she would have to undergo total knee replacement.

My friend was panicky. With help from me, he accessed another orthopaedic surgeon for a second opinion. The second specialist calmly explained that surgery is only the last resort in such cases. Even after knee surgery, the girl would have to keep on doing certain knee exercises for life. And if she does these exercises without undergoing surgery, she might never get her knee unlocked again, and hence might never require surgery. He explained that any surgery carries small but definite risks. His calm way of putting forth both alternatives was a contrast to the urgent threatening by the first surgeon.

Would we not like to opt for a doctor who does not create excessive fear or panic, but allows us to take properly informed decisions?

> **A rational, ethical doctor does not pretend to know everything; the doctor can admit that there are aspects of the illness that he or she cannot definitively comment upon.**

A fact which not all doctors might like to publicly admit is that in a significant number of cases, in the beginning, the doctor himself or herself may be unsure of the exact diagnosis. In these situations, the doctor is acting on probabilities rather than certainties. The doctor may rule out various possibilities only in the course of investigations and treatment. So when the patient or relative anxiously asks 'Doctor, what is the illness?', in a certain proportion of cases, the fact may be that even the doctor does not exactly know. This is inevitable given the unimaginable complexities of the human body, and the limits of medical knowledge. In such situations, the doctor may not be able to give a one-word answer, but instead of getting irritated at the patient (and at his own lack of certainty) the doctor needs to explain, at least in brief, the main probabilities and broad line of treatment. And regarding some questions, he or she might even have to muster the courage to utter the magic phrase which all doctors are conditioned to never speak—'I do not know'. It has been truly said that a wise man will admit what he does not know, while a fool cannot acknowledge his ignorance.

The importance of a doctor accepting the limits of his or her knowledge is emphasized by the following experience undergone by Dr Arun Gadre.

'One of the babies delivered at my hospital was suffering from a slight fever when it was just fifteen days old. The baby had been admitted under the care of a local general practitioner, who was sure that he could handle any case! The father was concerned about the treatment, and came to me with the request that I should visit the hospital to have a look at the baby. When I examined the baby, I felt that it was not as alert as expected, and might be having a serious problem. When I suggested shifting the baby to the care of a paediatrician, the general practitioner was furious. But the father followed my suggestion and shifted the baby to be cared for by a paediatrician. The baby was then diagnosed as being a very early case of meningitis (serious infection of the membranes surrounding the brain) but fortunately came out of this potentially life-threatening illness unscathed, due to early diagnosis and treatment!'

In these days of rapidly expanding medical knowledge, it is very difficult for any doctor to keep up with all the developments even in his or her own specialty, not to mention myriad other specialties and areas of medicine. Given this context, would we not prefer a doctor who is aware and frank about his or her own limitations, and who does not hesitate to take another expert opinion, or refer to another appropriate specialist, when required in the interest of the patient?

A rational, ethical doctor does not advise additional investigations and procedures, due to demands from the patient.

We live in a consumerist society, where we are often conditioned to think that 'more' is generally 'better'. If having a small car is good, a large car is better. If having some shoes is good, having a lot of shoes must be better. If having some wine is good, then having a lot of wine is better . . . . and so on. Needless to say this logic is often inappropriate, but some well-off patients tend to think that if undergoing some tests is necessary, then undergoing more investigations is even better, and if the test is more expensive, all the better!

However, the job of a physician is not to cater to each and every whim of the patient, but rather to guide the patient towards rational management of illness. Even though many laboratories give hefty commissions to doctors who refer patients to them (remember the testimonies in Part One of this book), a rational doctor would not recommend a test or procedure, just because the patient asks for it. Two experiences recounted here by Dr Gadre exemplify this.

'I was sitting beside my HIV specialist friend in his consulting room. A young chap had come for advice; he had a history of unsafe sex with a stranger just fifteen days back. He had already undergone his HIV test immediately afterwards. But he was very tense and was demanding one more HIV test and some more tests, there and then. My specialist friend did not succumb to his pressure. Instead of taking the simpler route of quickly writing a few tests, he took half an hour to counsel the young man. The patient became calmer and less anxious, and left with a smile on his face.

'I also remember another experience with a less positive outcome. A woman who was hardly thirty-five years of age had come to me, asking for her uterus to be removed. A general surgeon had done a plain X-ray of her abdomen (which usually cannot diagnose a condition like cancer in the uterus), and had alarmed her into thinking that she may have cancer of the uterus. The surgeon had advised her to undergo an emergency hysterectomy, supposedly to 'save her life'! She had panicked and come to me, asking for an operation to remove her uterus. I examined her and found that everything was normal. I did not succumb to her insistence, and counselled her. Alas, she was not convinced. Fear had gripped her, and she insisted on having her uterus removed. I was in a dilemma. If I disagreed with her, I would lose her as a patient, and someone else would go ahead and operate on her anyway! Yet I kept to my conviction and told her that I would not perform a procedure dictated by her fear. She went away, disappointed and was operated upon at some other hospital.'

How would you view a doctor who was willing to advise investigations or operations, just because one asked for it?

While these are some characteristics that we must look for in a doctor, we should also keep in mind that doctors are human beings who have to deal with very complex situations, often under considerable time pressure. Our expectations from a doctor should be tempered by an awareness of the kind of situations and unique challenges they often have to deal with; a few of these are mentioned here briefly, to complement the features we should look for while choosing a doctor mentioned above.[1]

Doctors often have to rely on information that is incomplete, while trying to understand what is wrong with the patient. Doctors continuously deal with uncertainty, and frequently work their way through the patient's illness, rather than always having an unambiguous diagnosis from day one.

This issue has been touched on above—the human body is an immensely complex entity which medical science understands only partially, and there are also tremendous variations from patient to patient. The information available to a doctor may be limited, and there may be unusual, unexpected or rare manifestations of an illness that the doctor must grapple with. While asking the doctor 'what is wrong with me?', we should be aware that sometimes the doctor may also not have the complete answer. Hence sometimes it may be more logical to talk in terms of possibilities and probabilities, rather than pressurizing the doctor to give a completely definitive answer. Such complexities faced by doctors while dealing with partial information are well illustrated by the following case experienced by Dr Gadre:

'The son of one of my relatives was admitted to the hospital with a sudden loss of consciousness, and was under the care of my physician friend. He was a young chap working in the IT industry, who was previously apparently normal, but had suddenly gone into a coma. My physician friend was clueless even after performing all the necessary tests. The consulting neurologist was also similarly confused. After three days of intensive treatment, the young man had not shown any improvement. My physician friend explained everything to me, including his inability to come to a diagnosis. A faint probability was that of tuberculosis, an omnipresent possibility in India! The physician suggested that we might try anti-tuberculosis drugs, while cautioning that they might prove to be completely useless. There was uncertainty and very limited information on which to take a decision. The father of the patient fully accepted the uncertainty, after receiving all related information from the physician. The 'trial' treatment for tuberculosis was started, and within four days the young man regained consciousness and then recovered without any problem.'

> **Good doctors continuously manage risk—doctors who are only interested in saving themselves may not save many patients.**

Many patients have survived and are living today, because the doctors treating them were willing to take certain risks. Especially doctors working in remote, rural and tribal areas know that recommending a critical patient be taken away to a distant city for treatment may be the equivalent of sending the patient home, and maybe to certain death. If it is within their sphere of competence, they may need to use their professional judgement and take informed and considered risks for the benefit of the patient. Of course doctors must never take reckless decisions or unjustified risks, or deal with matters that are beyond their competence. But a small risk taken by a doctor may make a huge difference and save a patient's life. Consider this experience of Dr Gadre:

'I was practising as a gynaecologist in a small town, without blood for transfusion being available. If I ordered a bottle of blood, it used to reach me from the nearest city 70 km away, after a gap of at least seven hours. And there was no public transport to the city after six in the evening.

'A woman in labour came to me at 8 o'clock at night, with her husband and her first kid, aged seven years. Her haemoglobin (an essential substance in the blood, whose level should be in the range of 12 to 15 grams) was just 6 grams. On examining her abdomen, I found that the elbow of the baby could be easily felt—this meant that her uterus had just ruptured; a very serious condition. If I tried to send her to the city, or waited to get blood from there, she would almost certainly die. I had to take the risk and operate on her, and conduct a caesarean to save her and her baby. But with her having just six grams of haemoglobin, and without blood available to transfuse her, I knew she was in a very risky situation, and I was in a serious dilemma. If things did not go well for her, she might not survive the operation. But where could she go? I explained everything to the husband who was a primary school teacher. He understood the magnitude of the risk I was undertaking, and the fact that at this point of time, she had no choice. He agreed, and both wife and husband gave their consent. I operated while being aware of the risk; fortunately both the mother and baby were saved. She did not require blood transfusion even while recovering.'

> **Doctors need to deal constantly with changing situations, both related to medical knowledge and society. They have to keep abreast of the rapidly changing field of medicine, and also grapple with the changing expectations of patients.**

The field of medical science is beset by new developments every month, and what was accepted practice even five years ago may have become obsolete now. At the same time, we need to keep in mind that many new drugs and investigations are being pushed by a highly commercialized industry, which might promote medicines and technologies that are not necessarily much superior or cost-effective, compared to the tried and tested existing ones. Doctors have to continually negotiate this maze of changing knowledge, and keep themselves updated. They need to choose treatments carefully, neither being swept away by each new technology, nor clinging to outdated methods, but rather choosing the optimal approach while placing the interests of the patient at the centre.

This complex situation becomes even more complicated due to the rapidly changing expectations of patients. Fortunately, today patients are on the whole better informed about illnesses and treatments than they used to be a generation ago; think of your overall awareness about health issues compared to, say, your parents. This positive change should be harnessed so that the doctor and patient/caregiver can work together as an informed team, in dialogue with each other, and choosing the best line of treatment that is appropriate to the patient. However, there is also a flip side to such increased awareness on medical issues. While Google has literally brought us a world of information, this information may not always be of uniformly high quality, or appropriate to the patient's specific situation. In some situations, patients may access half-baked and not entirely appropriate information off the internet, and may be firmly convinced that they need to undergo a particular line of treatment. How doctors need to deal with these significant and sometimes contradictory challenges, is well exemplified by two of Dr Gadre's experiences:

'The elderly lady gynaecologist had passed her sixties, but had a good practice. She had a thirty-nine-year-old woman who was taking antenatal care at her clinic, and this pregnant woman was also related to another, younger male gynaecologist. Most of the pregnancy passed without problem, and at thirty-six weeks of pregnancy (just a few weeks before expected delivery) the younger gynaecologist visited the patient and examined her. In just the previous week, the sonography had been normal. But when he examined the patient, the young gynaecologist felt that the fluid in the uterus, which surrounds and protects the baby, was a little less than expected—a situation that could be dangerous. He rang up the older gynaecologist and explained that he suspected a problem with the placenta, and would like to advise an urgent 'Colour Doppler' test (a special type of ultrasound test that is done in such cases); Colour Doppler. has been in use in India for more than fifteen years. Yet the older gynaecologist assured the younger one that she had a lot of experience; she felt that the baby was fine, and that there was no need for any further investigation.

'Fortunately the younger gynaecologist got the Colour Doppler test performed, and the investigation confirmed what he had suspected! There was very little fluid around the baby, who was now in serious danger. Within two hours, an emergency caesarean operation was performed at another hospital, and the baby survived after being resuscitated. The baby was saved in timely manner, thanks to the awareness of the younger gynaecologist about the newer technology and his knowledge about using it properly. Despite her considerable experience, the elderly gynaecologist had missed the bus, simply because she had not kept abreast with the changing methods of investigation in such situations.

'One of my orthopaedic surgeon friends narrated another case, which exemplifies the changing expectations of patients, and the emerging perils of 'Internetosis'. He was acquainted with an elderly couple in his city. The old woman was in her sixties and had mild arthritis. One day she visited him along with her husband. The old woman asked him to talk with their daughter living in the USA, who was an engineer. The daughter was aggressive with the orthopaedician over the phone, and complained that he was not doing his best to relieve her mother's suffering. She asked for the orthopaedician's email ID, as she wanted to send him some internet links related to knee replacement surgery. Money was not an issue, she asserted. She asked him to fix the date for knee replacement at least two months in advance, so that she could come to stay with her mother. The orthopaedician calmly and firmly explained that the old woman had mild arthritis, that pain killers were working well, and if the old woman were to take his advice seriously and start exercising as instructed, within two months even the pain killers could be stopped. In such a case, he asked, where is the need for total knee replacement? Though money was not an issue, there are issues like risk of anaesthesia, and infection in any surgery. Why choose surgery just because it is being promoted on some websites? He refused to operate and asked them to change the doctor if they felt like.

But the husband understood the doctor's logic, and two months later the old woman visited the orthopaedician with a bright smile. She had recovered completely, and had even stopped taking the pain killers. The knee exercises that had been advised had done a miracle. My orthopaedician friend commented: "Nowadays it is only rarely that I can convince a patient to change their mind, when the patient is educated, rich, and they have reached a decision after surfing the internet."

Four Kinds of Doctor–Patient Relationships

Finally, keeping in view all these aspects of how a doctor needs to function, it will be relevant to talk about the different ways in which doctors and patients relate with each other. In a classic paper,[2] Emanuel and Emanuel have described four kinds of doctor–patient relationships. The first one is the traditional relationship, which in India is probably still the most common. It could be termed as a 'Paternalistic' relationship—the doctor feels that he or she is the medical authority, and understands what is right for the patient ('The doctor knows best'). Given the perpetual asymmetry in knowledge, and also because the patient is often apprehensive about making an autonomous choice, doctors dispense advice, and patients are expected to follow it obediently. When a doctor is rational, empathetic, knowledgeable and ethical, many patients may not mind opting for this kind of relationship. But unfortunately today a significant number of doctors are abusing this relationship to generate fear and exploit patients, as the testimonies in the first part of this book reveal.

At the same time, people today have also become more aware and sensitive regarding their rights, and want to make choices related to treatment alternatives. Many are well informed and discerning; they would like all the relevant information, and then choose the option that seems best. In such situations, the Paternalistic relationship starts breaking down, and one alternative kind of relationship that emerges is called 'Informative'. This kind of approach is linked with the rise of 'informed consumers' in general. Information is central to modern living, and now, especially in developed countries, the medical profession has become accustomed to this kind of relationship. The doctor offers information about the choices that are available in a more or less neutral manner, and the patient makes the choices. This is, generally speaking, an advance over the Paternalistic approach, since patients today justifiably want information and control over decisions regarding their medical care.

However, patients want not just information, but also guidance. Merely reading about the survival percentages related to various options being offered does not offer much security to a patient who may be taking a crucial decision about their body, in a state of vulnerability. Even the most enlightened and empowered persons may not feel comfortable to take the entire responsibility of choosing between options, whose full implications may not be clear.

Dr Arun Gadre remembers the case of a noted literary person in Mumbai. 'He was advised angioplasty by a commercial cardiologist, just for slight muscular chest pain. I advised him to take a second opinion from a rationally practising, ethical cardiologist friend of mine. The second doctor told the patient that he need not even take a painkiller, since he was perfectly healthy; no intervention was required. A few months later, when I visited the eminent litterateur in Mumbai, he sheepishly told me that he had undergone an angioplasty as advised by the first cardiologist, because his family had decided not to opt for any risk. They feared: What if the second cardiologist, the rational one, was making a mistake?'

This happened in a non-emergency case, and to a highly educated and aware person. But what about an emergency, or the case of a less well-informed person? Would not the likelihood of being swayed by anxiety, and the inability to take a rational decision, have been even higher? In fact we all need not just information, but also interpretation and genuine advice. This requirement would never cease, however much bare information doctors may give us. Hence the relevance of a third type of doctor–patient relationship: 'Interpretive'. Here, the doctor does not order the patient as a paternalist, nor does he or she just stop after handing over the related information, waiting for the patient's decision. In this case the doctor helps the patient to articulate his or her values, and guides them to select the treatment that fits these values. The doctor makes the patient aware of their own value system, so that the patient can choose the treatment that matches this value system.

The interpretive approach undoubtedly has advantages compared to the first two approaches. But in this approach, the doctor does not have a dialogue with the patient regarding his or her value system, even though there may be significant issues related to this. For example, if a patient with heart disease is a workaholic, and wants to get cured as quickly as possible in order to get back to work, this kind of doctor may not enter into dialogue with the patient about the problems of being a workaholic. Hence the relevance of a fourth type of relationship—'Deliberative'—where the doctor and patient discuss not only the illness and treatment, but also touch upon the patient's value system, and the doctor tries to help the patient to refine his or her values, if felt appropriate. Where considered relevant, the doctor advises the patient not only on the treatment, but also on his or her broader approach. While in this approach the doctor engages more closely with the patient's values, it may be viewed as being intrusive by some.

Many of us may not be very happy with a strongly Paternalistic or purely Informative doctor–patient relationship. We may have some preferences for either a more Interpretive, or a more Deliberative relationship, or might like to have some combination. However we all know that when faced with pain, disability and perhaps even the dark shadows of mortality, we want not just 'instructions' or 'information', but we also need guidance, counselling and dialogue with our doctor. We need a doctor who would help us to interpret the complex mass of information around us, in the light of our internal values, to take an appropriate decision; we need a doctor who would deliberate with us and would help to bring out the best in ourselves, to choose the healthiest options in life, acting as a friend and guide, not just a detached expert.

Chapter 10

How Should the Private Medical Sector Be Regulated?

The reader would have gathered from the first part of this book, based on testimonies from various rationally practising, ethical doctors, that there is an urgent need to regulate the functioning of private hospitals and health care providers. Many of these doctors have emphasized the need for some kind of regulation to end the current anarchy in the private medical sector, so as to ensure rational, quality care. However, we need to keep in mind that in our country, the concept of 'regulation' has a mixed record in practice. Certain types of regulation have definitely helped to streamline and standardize specific sectors, such as the Telecom sector. Regulatory bodies like the Election Commission and the Comptroller and Auditor General (CAG) have helped to curb malpractices of certain types. But there are also several examples of top-down, bureaucratic and unaccountable regulation which contribute to corruption, without being of much benefit to the service users or general public. Further, in any regulatory framework, there is always the danger of 'elite capture', which means that the most powerful forces may hijack the entire regulatory process, and malpractices may continue, without much change in the situation for ordinary people. Keeping this context in mind, let us see how private hospitals can be effectively regulated in India, in the interests of common people and patients.

Self-regulation by the Medical Profession: The God That Failed
It has been said that the best form of discipline is self-discipline. In some ways, doctors are eminently well placed to effectively regulate the practices of their peers, since they have the expert knowledge and often intimate understanding of the practices of their colleagues, and they may be able to exert powerful peer pressure on anyone who tends to fall out of line. In several developed countries, the medical councils (bodies with legal authority composed mostly of doctors, and supposed to regulate doctors) are active in ensuring adequate standards of care and ethical conduct by doctors. The threat of de-registration by the Medical Council, barring the doctor from practising, can be one of the most potent threats to a doctor, reinforcing the motivation to practise ethically.

In the Indian context, the Medical Council of India (MCI) was supposed to ensure such self-regulation, at least at the level of ensuring ethical conduct by doctors. As mentioned in Chapter 8, the MCI has a detailed code of medical ethics, which is supposed to be followed by all doctors, and any doctor who is proven to not be following this code can be punished, even permanently de-registered. However, it is common knowledge that today unethical practices are rampant in the private medical sector in India, and the testimonies of our seventy-eight doctors reconfirms this unfortunate reality. Underlying this truth is the fact that doctors as a group have rarely spoken up about unethical practices by their colleagues. For example, the widespread and deeply condemnable practice of sex selection (leading to selective abortion of female foetuses) would be impossible, if doctors' associations were to publicly identify those among their vocation who indulge in such practices. And most State Medical Councils (which directly register doctors in various states) have rarely, if ever, taken proactive steps to identify and punish doctors indulging in unethical conduct.

For example, analysis of data related to the Maharashtra Medical Council, about disciplinary action being taken against doctors in the last decade (2005 to March 2015) shows that out of 746 complaints received against doctors, only 151 were decided upon, while the huge majority of 595 cases (nearly 80 per cent) were still pending. Out of those complaints that did get decided upon, some serious action was taken against the doctor in only three cases (out of 746 complaints), in the form of registration being temporarily withdrawn for three to six months.

It is interesting to note, that when moves for regulation of the private medical sector were initiated, and the central government began the formulation of a Clinical Establishments Act, certain doctors' associations were reminded of 'self-regulation' and started claiming that they did not need regulation by the state, since they were capable of regulating themselves. However, the sad reality is that the existing medical councils have by and large failed to ensure ethical conduct by doctors. And now regulation of the health sector cannot be left to doctors alone. Just like war is too important to be left to generals, the health care sector is too important to be left only to doctors, though obviously they would have an important role to play in any regulatory framework.

Problems with Traditional Bureaucratic Regulation, and Corporate-style Regulation[1]

Demanding regulation of the private health care sector and demanding its accountability are related concepts, but these are not necessarily identical. The experience of implementation of certain existing regulatory laws tells us that purely bureaucratic, top-down regulation, controlled by officials alone, may lead to 'red-tapism' (see the example of fire safety regulation in Chapter 5). Inspectors may focus on less important aspects of physical standards (like the type of tiles in a hospital room), while neglecting important process-related issues in the hospital. They may focus on a few trees and miss the forest. Such a limited regulatory system is also prone to breeding corruption; less scrupulous doctors may collude with inspectors, while honest doctors who refuse to 'satisfy' the inspectors may be harassed. Under such regulation, money may change hands frequently, but nothing much may change for the better in the hospital.

We also need to keep in mind that today there is intense competition in the private medical sector, and larger, corporate hospitals are trying to gain an increasing share of the 'market' (which in plain words means money from patients). One way of pushing out smaller hospitals with less resources is to shape the regulatory standards in such a manner that would favour big and well-resourced hospitals, who would be in a better situation to fulfil the legal standards. For example, if installing air conditioning in all hospitals were to become mandatory, then smaller hospitals with limited resources might be forced to shut down, or would have to overstretch themselves to meet the demanding standards.

Thus both purely bureaucratic regulation and corporate-hospital-oriented regulation would have their own limitations, since they may not reflect the concerns and experiences of patients and users of services. Such regulations may not be accountable to the ordinary people, whose interests they are supposed to protect. Both systems may also, in practice, tilt in the direction of larger and influential private hospitals at the expense of patients' interests, since the voice of the patients and ordinary people may not be represented in any form. In both kinds of systems, there is no social accountability of the regulators. So, do we have an alternative?

Social Regulation: Accountable, Participatory, Responsive

There is an alternative to 'non-regulation' of the private medical sector (mostly the current situation), as well as the above mentioned kinds of limited regulatory systems. That alternative would be a participatory, democratic regulatory system. In this kind of system, representatives of various concerned stakeholders (like elected representatives, public officials, representatives from the medical profession, consumer organizations, patients' rights groups) would interact in committees at district/city and state levels. These committees would oversee the work of inspectors and officials, they would discuss the various problems of patients as well as any doctors who might be aggrieved, and could prevent corruption in the regulatory process by means of such larger participatory oversight. The system of Health Councils in Brazil,[2] though not ideal, is a relevant positive example in this context. Multi-stakeholder bodies would evolve standards and norms, and officials along with technical experts would ensure their implementation. Citizens' organizations would monitor the fulfilment of patients' rights, and there would be people-friendly mechanisms to resolve any grievances. Since there would be oversight over the regulatory authorities by various stakeholders including citizens' groups, accountability of the regulatory structure is ensured. Democratic processes can prevent hijack of the regulators by powerful private interests. This model is informed by the understanding that regulation is actually a form of accountability, so regulators must be answerable to the wider public, within the framework of law.

Clinical Establishment Acts (CEAs)—What We Have, What We Need

Taking into view the entire context outlined until now, there is an urgent need for a legal framework that would effectively regulate the private medical sector in India. Fortunately, due to a variety of factors, today the need for such a framework has started coming on to the agenda, and at the centre of this is the move to enact 'Clinical Establishments Acts'.

To start regulating all types of hospitals and clinical establishments (which includes laboratories and diagnostic centres), the central government has passed a Clinical Establishments Act (CEA) in 2010, which has currently been adopted by several states (Rajasthan, Uttar Pradesh, Uttarakhand, Bihar, Jharkhand, Himachal Pradesh, Mizoram, Sikkim, Arunachal Pradesh and Assam) and all union territories. Some other states like Maharashtra and Kerala are also in the process of formulating similar acts. There are certain positive provisions in the central CEA, since this act:

- Makes display of rates by clinical establishments mandatory

- Lays down that rates have to be charged by clinical establishments in the defined, standard range
- Provides for standard treatment guidelines, which can ensure rational care
- Mandates registration of all clinical establishments (including laboratories and imaging centres), and covers all recognized branches of medicine (including Ayurveda and Homeopathy); it is not just restricted to modern medicine.

However, there two kinds of issues related to this national act. Firstly, while the act was passed in 2010, and the rules were adopted in 2012, the standards necessary for actual registration of hospitals are yet to be finalized as late as late 2015. Until the standards are finalized, the act cannot actually be implemented in any of the states where it is applicable. So progress on developing the supportive legal framework for this act has been rather slow, retarding its implementation until now. Secondly, there are certain gaps in the current national act which need to be rectified. As clarified above, there is a need for laws to regulate private hospitals that would be supported by social mechanisms, which could ensure transparent and accountable regulation, rather than just having bureaucratic regulations. Some of the key provisions that should be addressed in the legal framework at national level (these might be taken care of by modifying the rules, or could be included in the standards), and similar state-level acts, would be as follows:

- Ensure social regulation of the private medical sector. Even though most of the doctors we interviewed are in favour of regulation, many have suffered due to harassment by government officials. Therefore, many fear that any system of regulation might be used to promote corruption. However, many doctors are in favour of participatory regulation, where along with legal authorities, there is scope for an evidence-based review of decisions in a multi-stakeholder body, and both citizen and patient groups as well as doctors have forums for appeal. This implies that there should be an appellate board at the district level consisting of government officials, representatives of doctors, and health-related civil society organizations. One could review the decisions of regulatory officials in this appellate board based on concrete, appropriate evidence. This would curb arbitrary decisions, while ensuring compliance with the defined standards and rules.

- Another important aspect of the regulation of the private medical sector must be ensuring patients' rights (outlined in Chapter 8), standard treatment guidelines, and transparency as well as regulation concerning rates.

- Many doctors suspect that under the rubric of regulation, some corporate hospitals may be pushing for certain excessively demanding technical requirements (especially concerning infrastructure and equipment), which small hospitals cannot possibly meet. The state should take the Indian reality into consideration, and the valid concerns of small hospitals and patients must be kept in mind when bringing in any regulation. Many doctors emphasize that the standards under any system of regulation should not contribute to preferentially promoting corporate and large private hospitals.

- The framework must include an effective and people-friendly redressal mechanism to address the complaints of patients, as well as any grievances of doctors.

- Some doctors have stressed the need, while designing and operationalizing regulations, to take into consideration the valid concerns of genuinely charitable hospitals working in vulnerable, tribal and difficult areas with limited resources.

It may be added here that the practice of giving or taking cuts in medical practice must be legally prohibited. Similarly the sponsorship of doctors' conferences by pharmaceutical companies must be eliminated. If pharmaceutical companies want to sponsor CME (Continuing Medical Education) workshops, they should give funds to the Medical Association, without placing any conditions or having any intervention in organizing the workshop.

Medical Councils and Regulation of Private Medical Colleges: Need for 'System Upgrade'

We have noted above how self-regulation of the ethical conduct of doctors through various medical councils has been largely ineffective in our country. However, the problems with medical councils, including the Medical Council of India (MCI) at the national level, do not end here. Several of the doctors we interviewed expressed the view that today MCI needs major structural and functional reform. At present most of the members of MCI are government officials or doctors' representatives. Compared to the number of government officials, the number of patients' and civil society organizations' representatives need to be increased. The overall direction needs to be towards making the Council much more accountable, and oriented to the significant social concerns today regarding private medical colleges and the private medical profession.

It should also be noted here, on the positive side, that in some instances, medical councils have been proactive in taking steps to promote ethical conduct and public transparency by doctors. The Punjab Medical Council has publicly declared that all doctors and hospitals must display the rates of their services (as mandated by the Code of Medical Ethics). Also, the Medical Council of India has recently ruled that the licence to practice of fifteen senior doctors from Madhya Pradesh, who had taken foreign trips thanks to the 'hospitality' of pharmaceutical companies, should be suspended for six months as punishment.

However, such positive actions are still rare, and much, much more needs to be done by medical councils to prevent widespread unethical actions by doctors. Here, we also need to note briefly another hugely controversial area, which is also related to medical councils, namely the issue of private, 'donation'-based medical colleges.

Private, 'Donation'-based Medical Colleges

As noted by various doctors whom we interviewed (in Chapter 5, 'The Harmful Influence of Private Medical Colleges—Boon or Bane?'), medical colleges where students are forced to make huge 'donations'—in scores of lakhs and even crores, essentially to purchase medical degrees, have become increasingly common over the last two decades. On the one hand, there are serious allegations of corruption and public scams as well, with ongoing legal cases against certain senior and powerful office-bearers of the MCI, who are responsible for giving approval to such colleges. On the other hand, such colleges are driving extreme commercialization of medical care, since the doctors who graduate from these colleges often go to any extent of irrational and unnecessary procedures on a regular basis to 'recover' their 'investment'.

Given this situation, the fees being charged in all private medical colleges must be brought to the same level as those being currently charged in government medical colleges. No private medical college should be allowed to charge more than this norm. In addition, there should be a moratorium on starting new private medical colleges, at least for several years until the entire current mess has been cleaned up. Where genuinely required, the government should open its own new colleges with a view of training more doctors to work at the primary level, and to serve in the public health system. Overall, the current trend for increasing commercialization of medical education must be effectively curbed, and the trend of escalating costs of medical education must be reversed, if we want to ensure that the doctors being produced in our medical colleges—rather than being conditioned to become 'extortionists' driven by the compulsion for financial extraction—are groomed to practise as rational and ethical professionals, who keep the interests of patients at the centre.

Chapter 11

Moving towards a System for Universal Health Care (UHC)[1]

From the previous chapters, it would have become obvious to the reader that many of the current ills of the private medical sector in our country are linked to the increasingly commercialized nature of health care. When, instead of being a highly skilled and humane profession, health care becomes an arena for making investments and maximizing profits, then all kinds of distortions are bound to emerge. Suppliers begin to artificially boost the demand; doctors define which procedures patients should undergo, and recommend unnecessary ones—just like if barbers were to decide if people needed a haircut, they would advise cropping everyone's hair! Unhealthy, cut-throat competition promotes malpractices like the system of commissions and kickbacks. While regulation of standards and protection of patients' rights are important first steps to address this situation, we progressively need to create a system that will ensure the relations between doctor and patient no longer remain a buyer-seller relationship. Patients should not have to pay doctors for their services, and doctors should not have to charge patients to make an income, which is possible if both are part of a publicly organized and financed system.

Such a publicly organized system is called 'Universal Health Care' (not to be confused with the similar term Universal Health Coverage, which is usually linked with commercial health insurance). Today, UHC systems exist in Canada, Australia, Brazil, Thailand, the UK and several European countries. In these countries, public health services, trust hospitals and private hospitals have been engaged in a publicly managed system, which provides free health care to the entire population. Large sections of the private medical sector have been absorbed into the system, and a public body pays and regulates the hospitals and doctors on behalf of the patient. In such a system, decisions related to treatment are not based on how much money the patient can pay, rather everyone has access to a standard quality of health care. The public body takes the responsibility to ensure provision of health services, which is supported mainly through taxes while in some countries it is supplemented by social insurance.

This scenario may appear unrealistic to Indian readers, but following on the examples of developing countries like Thailand and Brazil, today if there is sufficient political and social will, an appropriate UHC system can be implemented in India. This would put a major brake on profiteering and commercialization of health care, since rates for all services would be standardized, and health care would be largely removed from the vagaries of the market. Such a system would ensure access to rational (neither excessive nor deficient) health care for all sections of the population, and could ensure a decent and stable income for doctors without the continuous pressures of competition, while eliminating the commercialized environment that breeds irrational care, violation of patients' rights and commission practice.

Let us start the discussion on this approach with a real-life story, and then explore through a series of questions and answers what a UHC system means and entails, and how such a system could be realistically developed in India.

The accident happened on 7 October 2006. Narin fell off his motorcycle while turning into a bend. He struck a tree, his unprotected head taking the full force of the impact. Passing motorists found him some time later and took him to a nearby hospital. Doctors diagnosed severe head injury and referred him to the trauma centre, 65 km away, where the diagnosis was confirmed. His skull had fractured in several places. A scan showed that his brain had bulged and shifted, and was still bleeding; the doctors decided to operate. He was wheeled into an emergency department where a surgeon removed part of his skull to relieve pressure. A blood clot was also removed. Five hours later, the patient was put on a respirator and taken to the intensive care unit where he stayed for twenty-one days. Thirty-nine days after being admitted to hospital, he had recovered sufficiently to be discharged.

What is remarkable about this story is not what it says about the power of modern medicine to repair a broken body; it is remarkable because the episode took place not in a 'developed' or 'rich' country, where annual per capita expenditure on health care is very high, (close to US$ 4000 or around Rs 2.5 lakh), but in Thailand, a country that spends only about one-thirtieth of this amount (US$ 136 or around Rs 8000) per capita on health. For Thailand, this amounts to just 3.7 per cent of its gross domestic product (GDP). Nor did the patient belong to the ruling elite, the type of person who tends to get good treatment wherever they live. Narin was a casual labourer, earning only US$ 5 a day.

'Thai legislation demands that all injured patients be taken care of with standard procedure no matter what their status,' says the surgeon who operated on Narin. The surgeon further clarified that medical staff do not consider who is going to pay for treatment, however expensive it might be, because in Thailand, everyone's health care costs are covered.

(Source: WHO, 2010, 'The World Health Report, Financing for Universal Coverage')

We would naturally ask, what does it mean when Narin's surgeon says 'everyone's health care costs in Thailand are covered'? Is it possible to pay for health care in advance, and not have to pay while seeking care? And who actually pays for the care when the surgeon says 'it is paid for'? Was the hospital being referred to a public or private hospital? Is it possible that doctors will directly start treatment without asking for an advance in a private hospital? Is such a system possible in India? Let us try to discuss such a system by answering some major questions.

1. What Do We Mean by a System for 'Universal Health Care'[2] (UHC)?

'Universal Health Care' means a system which aims to provide the entire population of a country good quality health services according to needs and preferences, regardless of income level, social status, or place of residence.

The term 'universal' means the entire population. Every citizen and resident of the country is covered by the respective services; such a system serves not only the entire spectrum of rural and urban poor, but also the middle class and better-off sections of society.

In a system for Universal Health Care, services would be as follows:

- **Good quality services** would include a comprehensive package of preventive services, outpatient care, hospitalization services and rehabilitative care—all the essential services required for a healthy life. However, this may initially not include certain very expensive treatment options, or non-essential services like cosmetic surgery for 'beautification'. Every attempt must be made to include all important forms of health care and treatment options within the fold of UHC, making them accessible to all.

- **According to needs and preferences** means that all the people needing services would be covered and that the neediest will be prioritized. Secondly, people will have reasonable choice about their treatment options, such as whether to take treatment from an Ayurvedic provider or allopathic provider, and choice between a range of therapies available for that ailment in the given UHC framework.

- **Regardless of income level** means irrespective of the person's ability to pay, even the poorest will be able to access the full spectrum of provided services.

- **Regardless of social status** means marginalized social groups such as dalits, adivasis, minority communities or other vulnerable groups such as single or deserted women, orphans, elderly, disabled, migrants and others will have equal access to this package of health care.

- **Regardless of place of residence** means the current inequality between urban and rural areas, or across different regions would be overcome to ensure quality care to all needy people, including those in rural and remote areas.

2. Why Is It Necessary to Have a System for Universal Health Care in India?

For readers who have gone through all the previous chapters of this book, and who are acquainted with the current health care situation in India, this may seem to be a rather silly question, whose answer is obvious. However, let us briefly go over some major arguments:

- The majority, i.e. around 80 per cent of outpatient care and 60 per cent of hospitalization care in India, is provided by the private medical sector. Today there are practically no controls or checks and balances regarding the quality, price or rationality of private health care services.

- Due to problems of insufficient funding, understaffing and insufficient accountability, the network of public health services is below expectation in availability and quality of services, as well as concerning responsiveness to the patients. The present scale of public health services is inadequate to cater to the needs of the entire population—rural and urban, poor and well-off, basic and advanced care.

- Given this situation, and the fact that various types of health care protection (such as insurance) are limited or inadequate, most patients have to pay from their own pockets for health services, and they often undergo 'catastrophic' health care spending.

The consequences of this, especially for those who cannot pay, are as follows:

- **Frequent impoverishment on account of health care:** Around half of the households where a member undergoes hospitalization have to borrow money or sell ornaments and other assets to meet hospitalization-related expenses. Every year, about 3.5 crore Indians are pushed into poverty due to health care expenses.

- **Extreme inequities in access to health care:** There are massive inequities in health services availability across the country, and across social classes. These inequities in access to health care are growing, and are adding to the larger social and economic inequities in the country.

- **Irrationalities and wastages:** As documented throughout this book, a serious problem with our unregulated and largely privatized health care set-up is irrational and wasteful care. To give an example, caesarean section rates among well-off women are seventeen times higher as compared to poor women. The rich, urban women are undergoing an irrationally high number of caesarean sections while the poor, rural women often do not have access to essential caesarean operations even when genuinely needed.

This entire situation—which may be justifiably regarded as a crisis situation for ordinary people—calls for organizing a more affordable, equitable, rational and efficient health care system, all of which can be ensured through a system for Universal Health Care.

3. What Would Be the Principles and Core Elements of the UHC System?[3]

As we shall see in this chapter, various countries have used varying strategies to ensure universal access to health care; some have been more successful than others. The principles for any UHC system would be those core values which allow us to assess if progress is being made in the right direction. The following are such principles:

- **Universality:** As the name suggests, it is important that all residents of the country be covered under UHC. UHC should not be restricted to any population group such as only the formal employees, or those who can pay and contribute, or only those who are 'below poverty line'.

- **Equity and non-discrimination:** A UHC system should be fair and egalitarian. This means that it must be available to all, irrespective of class, caste, gender and social background or geographical location. However, care for the medically neediest may be prioritized, such as those with more serious illnesses or where time-bound treatment, as in case of an emergency, will make a huge difference.

- **Comprehensive care:** The range of services available in a UHC system should be as broad as possible to meet the entire range of health care needs, taking into account the local patterns of illnesses and needs of different sections of the population, including vulnerable sections. Every effort should be made to ensure the spectrum of essential services, and to include the use of cost-effective technology.

- **Financial protection:** UHC should guard against impoverishment of people on account of health care expenses.

- **Quality and rationality of care:** UHC should ensure prescribed quality and standards of care and should follow guidelines for rational care. UHC is not about providing more and more health services to people, but is about ensuring that only rational and appropriate health care is provided.

- **Portability and continuity of care:** Treatment for an illness should not be discontinued when the patient changes residence. This is relevant in the case of migrant workers, pregnant women who decide to deliver at their natal homes etc. Emergency care must be available to all, including those who travel to any place in the country. There should be no gap in care when patients are transferred from one facility to another.

- **Protection of patients' rights, appropriate care, and patients' choice:** UHC should be designed to protect patients' rights (described in Chapter 8) such as right to information, informed consent, right to confidentiality and privacy etc. A grievance redressal system should be in place in case the patient or caregivers have complaints.

- **Participation, transparency and accountability:** This would ensure that people are involved at various stages of planning and monitoring of UHC. People would be informed and can ask questions, demand redressal of any grievances, and the system will be accountable to them. The health councils in Brazil and health assemblies in Thailand are examples of processes to ensure accountability of UHC systems.

- **Consolidated and strengthened public health provisioning:** Provision of services by strengthened public facilities would be at the core of the UHC system. Public bodies should play the coordinating role in deciding the roles and responsibilities of all facilities, including the private sector, in provisioning under the UHC system.

- **Central role of public financing:** The prime responsibility of financing the UHC system should be with the state—through public financing, primarily general taxes. This would also mean that the doctors and hospitals would be paid from a single pool of funds, and patients will not have to pay anything at the point of service. Health care is a human right, and nobody should be denied health care on the grounds of inability to pay fees for health care. In UHC systems in both developed and developing countries, there is generally no payment or hardly any payment to be made by the patient at the point of service. Most of the health care expenses are met through a consolidated pool of funds. Such a 'single-payer mechanism', based on general taxation, is equitable, because the poor have as much right as the rich to get health care, though their contribution to taxes may be lower.

4. Has Any Country Been Able to Ensure UHC for Its People?

UHC is not a fairy tale, although at first glance it may appear to be so. Many countries have been able to ensure UHC for their residents. Most European countries have ensured UHC for their citizens during the last sixty years. Prominent examples are the National Health System of the United Kingdom, UHC models of Scandinavian and west European countries such as France, Germany and the Netherlands. Health care systems of Canada and Australia are also other leading examples of UHC among the non-European countries. USA is a notable negative exception, where despite very high health care spending, citizens do not enjoy universal access to health care, and about 50 million (20 percent) of US citizens do not have health care protection. Under the Obama-led administration, some partial efforts are being made to address this situation in the US,[4] but these do not amount to a single-payer UHC system.

What is more relevant for people in India is that several low- and middle-income countries have also achieved UHC systems. Some Asian examples are:

- **Thailand:** Thailand introduced UHC in 2001. This South East Asian country has nearly 60 per cent of its population residing in rural areas. It has a large private medical sector, and the majority of workers are in the informal sector. Their earlier issues of health care access were similar to the ones seen currently in India. After the introduction of UHC in 2001, the population having health care protection reached 98.7 per cent by the year 2004. In 2006, the Thai government made access to UHC completely free of charge by abolishing the copayment of 30 baht (about Rs 57), which was required to be paid earlier by patients for every visit to the doctor.

- **Sri Lanka:** Our southern neighbour, Sri Lanka, started the expansion of a strong public health system as early as 1931, with the election of its first democratic government. This expansion was done by increasing the government's budget for health care. Today, Sri Lanka provides free primary and secondary health care, including free medicines for all residents through the public health system. It also has a strong preventive and promotive health care component, excellent awareness of health rights and a very good public health response to emergencies as seen at the time of the tsunami. As a result, various health indicators of this middle-income country compete with the developed countries.

- **Republic of Korea** and **Malaysia** are other countries in Asia that have been able to institute a system for Universal Health Care and cover most of their population.

Some Latin American countries have also achieved UHC. **Cuba** is a notable example, which achieved UHC within a few years of its revolution in 1962, entirely through public provisioning of health care. The Cuban health care system is considered to be one of the best in the world, which ensures health outcomes comparable to most developed countries, but at a fraction of their cost.

Brazil is the fifth largest country in the world, and has tremendous geographical diversity and significant socio-economic inequities, similar to India. The 1988 Brazilian Constitution made access to health care a universal right, and developed the 'Unified Health System', a national system to deliver health care. This system includes, apart from all public facilities, those private facilities which accept the terms of UHC, thus bringing private hospitals under a public system. Today, everyone in Brazil has the right to use health services in the country at no out-of-pocket cost.

More recently **Venezuela** has taken important steps towards Universal Health Care, through very effective systems of public provisioning focused on primary health care, based on an innovative programme of neighbourhood primary care clinics called 'Barrio Adentro' (translated from Spanish this roughly means 'inside the low-income neighbourhood').

Even though the current political systems in some of the mentioned countries provide a very different context from the present situation in India, we can learn valuable lessons from their initiatives in the health care sector.

5. How Are UHC Systems Financed?

Thailand and Brazil have Universal Health Care systems, where the level of public health expenditure required to support such systems is 3.7 per cent and 4.7 per cent of the GDP respectively. In the Indian context, it has been estimated that putting in place a UHC system may require an investment of at least around 4 per cent of the GDP. Overall, developing a UHC system in India would imply a significant increase in the scale of public health finances. The two main routes to finance a system of UHC in any country are through taxes and social health insurance.

- **Direct and indirect taxation:** This is the most cost-effective and equitable means of raising finances for UHC. It is cost-effective because it requires less administrative mechanisms. It is equitable because direct taxation is generally in proportion to income, and thus more contribution is collected from the higher-income groups. For example, in

Thailand and Brazil general tax funding makes up the major share of the financing for UHC.

India has used special tax as a method to finance certain essential services, e.g. an education cess of 3 per cent is applicable on income, in order to finance basic education. Higher taxes for luxury items and taxes on disease-causing items like tobacco and alcohol, which are inherently deleterious to health, can also enhance resources for UHC.

- **Social Health Insurance:** In a typical health insurance scheme, all those who are enrolled pay a premium in advance. Then the bills of those who might fall ill are paid (within an upper limit) through this pool of funds, created through advance payment. Hence, in any insurance mechanism, the risk of falling ill and need for medical treatment is pooled on a mandatory basis among a group.

Social Health Insurance, Commercial Insurance (provided by insurance companies) and Community Health Insurance are some major methods of insurance. Of these three, Social Health Insurance is much more progressive, equitable and inclusive in nature. Countries such as Germany in Europe, and Japan and Republic of Korea in the Asia-Pacific region have a Social Health Insurance-based UHC system. However, it should be noted that there is no comprehensive UHC system in the world based on private insurance or community-based insurance alone.

Countries that have UHC systems based on Social Health Insurance generally have a social insurance fund covering almost the entire population, where contributions from employers, employees, the self-employed and the government are pooled. In this system, the government steps in to contribute for those who do not have the resources to pay insurance premiums. Though more equitable than private insurance, Social Health Insurance-based health care is generally less cost-effective than tax-financed options, and is associated with greater administrative costs.

6. Can Private Health Insurance Be the Basis for a UHC System?

In no country in the world has private health insurance been the primary basis for comprehensive UHC. In some countries, such as the United States, people mainly use private insurance to ensure access to health care, but this results in major problems. As mentioned above, a large section of the population is not covered, or is inadequately covered by insurance. Experience has shown that private insurance is not a good mechanism for health care protection of an entire population because:

- Profit maximization is the stated goal of the private insurance companies. This leads to a tendency to reject claim payments, even if they are legitimate medical expenses.
- There are multiple insurance companies and schemes. Therefore the health system is fragmented and it is difficult to regulate or make guidelines for the system.
- Due to multiple providers and litigation owing to rejected claims, the administrative costs, litigation costs, inefficiencies and wastages of the system tend to be quite high.

Overall, in the Indian context, while individual families may today opt for commercial insurance (in the form of schemes like Mediclaim), in the absence of any other form of protection, it is clear that commercial insurance cannot become the basis of a comprehensive UHC system. Taking individual health insurance today is a stopgap measure that many middle-class people resort to, because there is no larger, publicly organized system to protect the entire population. It is a bit like drinking bottled water, since we perceive the public water supply to be unsafe. Rather than encouraging everyone to buy and drink bottled water, it would be much more rational and cost-effective to ensure that an improved public water supply system delivers safe drinking water to everyone.

7. Who Provides Services in a UHC System? Does the Patient Have to Pay for Services When Going to the Doctor?

There are two major models of health care provisioning seen in UHC systems—public provision of services, and mixed public–private provision of services.

- **Mostly public provisioning of health care services:** Most well-functioning UHC systems have a significant component of public health provisioning. Further, in some UHC systems, much of the primary care and also the commonly required secondary care are provided free of cost by public dispensaries and hospitals, e.g., Sri Lanka. In such systems, where public provisioning is dominant, the private sector may be contracted in to provide services only where public services do not exist (e.g., specific areas), or for relatively less common problems (e.g., super-specialized services). They provide services on terms set by the public system and under public regulation, thus effectively being an extension of the public system.

- **Public and private mixed provision of services:** Many countries with UHC systems provide health care through a mixture of public and private providers. They have either a public or an autonomous institution which decides the terms of purchase of services, fees for various services, standards of care and terms for provisioning services, thus regulating this system. In each area some public and private facilities are designated for care. However, it may not be possible to directly approach a specialist doctor, and one may have to go through the organized referral system. Public and private providers together form the UHC provisioning system.

Here it should be emphasized that in the Indian context, any kind of UHC system would require significant strengthening and expansion of public health services, improving their quality and responsiveness, while putting in place vibrant systems for social accountability at all levels. An adequately resourced, well-functioning and responsive public health system needs to be the backbone of the UHC system, and can prove to be a strong counterbalance and check on commercialization of health care by the private medical sector. This is clearly demonstrated by many examples such as Sri Lanka and Indian states like Mizoram and Goa, which have well-developed public health systems.

It should also be noted here that UHC in the Indian context should include AYUSH (Ayurveda, Yoga and Naturopathy, Unani, Siddha, Homeopathy) systems of healing as an option at various levels of health care. We can draw upon the positive experiences of China, which has effectively integrated modern medicine and traditional Chinese medicine. So far in India, AYUSH systems have received discriminatory treatment from the government. However, AYUSH should have a rightful place in UHC. This would consist of provision, at all levels of AYUSH, of measures that are effective and safe; such provisioning would enable us to move towards an integrated approach to health care.

Whether primarily publicly provided, or provided through a mix of public and private providers, the services given to patients in a UHC system should generally be free of cost, since the health care providers are paid from public finances. UHC systems in some countries have introduced elements of 'copayment', which means that patients need to pay small amounts for certain facilities and goods, which is not a desirable feature. This should be avoided by raising finances for the UHC system through public means.

8. How Can People Ensure that the UHC System Is Accountable, and that It Delivers Services As Expected?

Many people in India are sceptical about publicly organized services, since these may not be sufficiently accountable and responsive. But public services and systems can function well, if on the one hand they are well resourced and staffed, and on the other hand there are effective systems for accountability and people's participation in ensuring their proper functioning. Keeping this context in mind, any UHC system must include mechanisms for accountability and participation of citizens and social organizations, to ensure that the system meets the needs of its users, and it effectively responds to any gaps or problems that may be experienced by people.

The system of Health Councils in Brazil is a good example of how social groups and citizens' organizations can be involved in making a UHC system accountable and responsive. Brazil has set up over 5000 participatory committees called health councils across the country, at three levels—national, state and municipal levels (the municipal level is similar to an Indian taluka). One-fourth of the members of each health council are from the government and health care providers, one-fourth are representatives of health professionals and employees, while half of the members are health service users and consumer groups. The health councils are powerful bodies mandated with health planning and monitoring the functioning of the UHC system. This fosters people's active participation and accountability to users. Further, 'health conferences' are held at various levels across the country every few years, where hundreds and even thousands of citizens and representatives of social groups meet and brainstorm to shape and plan the UHC system in Brazil, thereby ensuring that it remains responsive to people's needs.

In Thailand, there is a system of organizing 'health assemblies' at the national level on an annual basis, to ensure large-scale social participation in shaping the UHC system, while making it responsive. The assembly comprises three groups: representatives from government or politicians, representatives from academic and expert groups, and representatives from various social organizations. Such participatory processes increase awareness among the general public on health issues, and provide a platform for people to present points, which the UHC system should address.

In the Indian context, Community Based Monitoring and Planning (CBMP) of health services, which has been effectively developed on a pilot basis in a few states like Maharashtra,[5] is an effort towards making health services accountable to community members, while promoting their involvement in local planning processes. CBMP, a tool introduced as part of the National Rural Health Mission[6] on a pilot basis in certain districts of some states, enables ordinary people to audit health services for satisfactory performance. The observed gaps and people's expectations are then communicated to the health officials in 'jan sunwais' (public hearings) as well as through dialogue in participatory committees. Such experiences, and processes like participatory planning in Kerala, and communitization of health services in Nagaland, can be built upon, while devising accountability and participation mechanisms for a UHC system in the Indian context.

9. WHAT IS NOT A SYSTEM FOR 'UNIVERSAL HEALTH CARE'?

In the above sections, we have tried to briefly understand what constitutes a system for Universal Health Care, drawing upon experiences in certain other countries. However, different experts and agencies have a varying understanding of what is actually meant by a system for Universal Health Care, and many experts use the similar sounding term, 'Universal Health Coverage'. These are somewhat different concepts, which are associated with different kinds of models and methods to organize health care. Here, we will clarify, in our understanding what is not a system for 'Universal Health Care', though certain existing schemes may have some superficial resemblance to the concept of UHC.

Currently, the Arogyasri Health Scheme in Andhra Pradesh is being quoted by some expert bodies as a major step towards 'Universal

Health Coverage'. This scheme facilitates government-funded health care to patients below a particular income level (constituting around 80 per cent of the population). People have been enabled (originally through mediation by an insurance company) to obtain certain selected, specialized services (mostly operations or specialized treatment of certain complicated conditions). These may be provided by either public or private providers on a cashless basis, up to a limit of Rs 1.5 lakh in a year. Similar schemes have been initiated and are now in various stages of implementation in Tamil Nadu, Karnataka, Maharashtra and some other states. At another level, the Rashtriya Swasthya Bima Yojana (RSBY) covers 'below poverty line' (BPL) families in most states of India, by offering health insurance coverage up to Rs 30,000 per year for a family, for basic hospitalization care.

While these kinds of government-supported health coverage schemes (mostly operated through commercial insurance companies) may provide some relief to people, related to limited types of hospital-based care, we would state that in their current form they do not constitute a system for Universal Health Care. We may keep in mind:

- Mere provision of an insurance card for health care does not constitute a system for Universal Health Care. Just providing subsidized insurance cover, while letting the health care system (especially private providers) continue to function in an unregulated manner without rational care guidelines, rational fee structure, minimum standards, observance of patients' rights and other criteria mentioned as UHC principles (noted in Question 3 of this section) are not sufficient to develop a system for Universal Health Care. Private hospitals may be few in precisely those areas (remote, tribal or hilly areas) where the public health provisioning is also weak, so just giving people a card may not be the same as ensuring health care for them. Further, providing large-scale public funds to unregulated and not-very-rational private hospitals may lead to a spurt in unnecessary medical procedures. The 'epidemic' of hysterectomies in Andhra

Pradesh, facilitated by the Arogyasri scheme, is an example of this (following public outcry, hysterectomy has been removed from the list of services given by private hospitals under this scheme). Similarly, large-scale unnecessary hysterectomies have been performed in states like Chhattisgarh and Bihar, as part of the RSBY scheme.

• Providing selective forms of specialized health care, as seen in the Arogyasri scheme, which tends to channelize public funds towards delivery of specialized operations and advanced care, while ignoring basic health services, cannot be considered a system for Universal Health Care. In fact, such schemes tend to push people into hospitalization-based care, rather than promoting health and strengthening basic health care.

• Providing targeted care, catering only to the BPL section of the population (as is the situation with the RSBY scheme), also does not constitute a system for Universal Health Care.

10. WOULD ACCESS TO HEALTH CARE BE SUFFICIENT TO ENSURE BETTER HEALTH FOR PEOPLE?

Providing the full range of essential health services to all through a UHC system is quite important, but this alone cannot ensure an optimal standard of health for the entire population. Health is dependent not only on the provision of health care, but is also crucially linked with healthy living conditions, dietary intake and environment. Hence moving towards the goal of 'Health for All' requires, along with a system for UHC, also a provision of key health-related factors such as food security, nutrition, water supply, sanitation, healthy environmental conditions etc.

Keeping this in mind, while working for a UHC system, we must be aware of the risk of a highly medicalized model of care. If an over-medicalized approach to health care (which dominates much of the private sector in India today) prevails while developing a UHC system, this would only focus on ways to provide the latest health care technology to all, but may not check the factors which generate ill health. For example, such a medicalized approach may provide a vaccine for diarrhoea, but may not advocate for improving water supply and sanitation. Thus, conditions causing ill health would continue, illnesses would continue to be widely prevalent, and health care costs would keep increasing. To avoid such a situation, it is important that along with the UHC system, the state and society must also work for disease prevention and health promotion. This may include, along with providing the entire range of public services related to health, the development of community initiatives for improved nutrition, control of tobacco, alcohol and drug consumption, and developing widespread public awareness regarding healthy lifestyles and diet.

11. What Would Be a Suitable Model for Financing a UHC System in India? Can Our Government Raise the Necessary Scale of Funds?

As mentioned above, tax-based UHC systems are known to be the most equitable and efficient basis for a UHC system—examples being the UK, Brazil, Thailand and Sri Lanka. Hence India must strive for general as well as specific taxation to fund a UHC system. For this, central and state governments would need to combine their efforts. The government is already committed to increasing health care expenditure to 3 per cent of GDP, which is likely to be adequate for initiating a UHC system. If required, further funds can be raised by ending subsidies to the commercial private medical sector, and by imposing a health cess on health-damaging industries such as tobacco, alcohol and polluting industries. This might be supplemented by Social Health Insurance for employees in the organized sector and taxpayers, but all funds should be integrated into a single pool with a single-payer mechanism.

Today there is ample evidence about the hardships, impoverishment and misery that is the fate of millions of people in India on account of inadequate access to health care. Governments can raise the resources, as well as put in place the system, but what is lacking today is a strong social demand for a system of Universal Health Care. If there is widespread social demand for such a system, various political parties would raise the issue and the government would have to respond.

12. What Can We Do to Further This Demand, and Move Towards UHC in India?

Indeed, all of us can contribute to making UHC a reality in India. Those of us who are part of organized groups such as employees' associations, consumer organizations, unions, neighbourhood associations, women's groups, etc. can ensure that UHC starts becoming a demand from all of these groups. A well-thought-out system of UHC should become a strong social demand, while avoiding half-baked populist medical insurance schemes. Whatever kind of UHC system is proposed, it must take into account the needs and rights of all groups in society, including vulnerable and marginalized sections. Some first steps that can be taken in the immediate future, which would pave the way for a system for UHC in India, include the following:

- **Significantly strengthen the public health system while making it accountable:** Currently the public system caters to only about one-fourth of people's health care needs. It is also perceived to be bureaucratic and non-responsive to people's needs. The public health system needs to be strengthened with infusion of funds, infrastructure and human power, since it would be the backbone of the UHC system. Simultaneously it needs to be made accountable and its functioning has to become more effective and responsive to people, through measures such as Community Based Monitoring and Planning (CBMP).

- **Regulation of private medical providers:** As discussed in the previous chapter, private hospitals, nursing homes and other clinical establishments need to be regulated and standardized to ensure minimum standards of care, rationality of care, reasonable fees, patients' rights and a grievance redressal mechanism. Towards this, standard guidelines for quality of care, treatment protocols and rational cost estimates of common health care services need to be developed. Trust hospitals, which have availed of large-scale public subsidies in terms of land at minimal cost and other benefits, must be made to effectively provide 20 per cent of beds for economically-weaker sections.

- **Substantially increase public health financing:** India is already committed to increasing health financing to 3 per cent of GDP from the current level of 1.2 per cent. This implies making a quantum jump in the health care budget, a significant part of which should be utilized for strengthening of the public health system and enhancing health sector human power, while developing frameworks for regulating the private medical sector in parallel.

- **Ensuring laws and governance for the health system:** Enactment of a National Health Act, which ensures the right to health and health care for all, could be an important legal step. Community Based Monitoring should be extended to ensure participatory planning and monitoring of all health services, with active involvement of civil society organizations. Generating widespread awareness and people's organization for health rights is an essential condition to make any UHC system in India work successfully in people's interest.

The dozen questions and answers above should give the reader an overall idea about a system for UHC, and how this goal can be achieved in India. Though it may sound like a dream, given the experience of so many other countries, it is clear that UHC is a realizable dream. In the early twenty-first century, for both people and doctors, health care should cease to be a commodity, and should become a publicly organized service. With such a framework, health care should be considered a human right. Starting from the present crisis situation, moving towards a system which would fulfil the health rights of all residents in India, and would provide a stable, decent income with healthy working environments for all doctors, is a stupendous challenge, and would require extensive social churning. It is high time that all of us rise to meet this challenge, and convert the dream of Universal Health Care into reality.

Chapter 12

Joining Hands for Healing the Health Sector

In the pages of this book, we have seen how a significant number of practising doctors have alerted us about the massive distortions that have come to pervade the private medical sector. We have also gone over some possible directions by which we can move out of this morass, including the promotion of patients' rights, identifying and opting for rational, ethical doctors, effectively regulating the private medical sector, and developing a system for Universal Health Care.

In this concluding chapter, we will focus on some collective measures and social processes that can be taken up to deal with the crisis in the health sector, keeping in mind the analyses outlined in the previous chapters. Asserting rights as a patient or caregiver in a private hospital (Chapter 8) and choosing a rational, ethical doctor (Chapter 9) can be done to some extent, on an individual basis. But it may not always be feasible to identify and access rational doctors in our area through individual efforts—this may require more cooperative efforts, which have been suggested here. We will also see how we can collectively work for much-needed policy changes in the health sector, which have been outlined in some of the previous chapters. It would also be relevant to reflect upon our existing attitudes towards health, and discuss if we need some changes in the increasingly consumerist social ethos related to health and health care in India.

Developing 'Citizen–Doctor Forums'

Today, due to the large-scale commercialization of health care, there is widespread confusion, distrust and suspicion, and an uneasy relationship frequently prevails between private health care providers and patients. The asymmetry of information (and consequent power) is profound; being aware of this fact, patients often feel vulnerable and helpless. When one is a patient, he or she may have very little leeway to negotiate and make choices, since many doctors (barring some notable exceptions) operate in a 'paternalistic' mode. In Chapter 9, we have discussed the features of a rational, ethical doctor, but the reality is that when required, it may not be easy for an ordinary patient to identify and locate such doctors, in the specialty and geographical area required.

Regarding hospitals and laboratories, there is a system of accreditation (facilitated by bodies like National Accreditation Board for Hospitals & Health Care Providers (NABH) and National Accreditation Board for Testing and Calibration Laboratories (NABL) which mostly focuses upon the infrastructural and procedural standards of the hospital or laboratory. While such accreditation serves some purpose, by encouraging basic standards in clinical establishments, it does not deal with issues of rationality of care and ethicality of practice by individual doctors. Hence the vulnerable patient does not know how to search for a good doctor, except by 'word of mouth' and personal contacts. In today's world, with the growing complexity of health care, large-scale individual mobility and weakening of community ties, such personal means are not sufficient.

We should note that there is a problem here not only for patients, but also for rational, ethical doctors. On the one hand, certain corporate hospitals and large multi-specialty hospitals are luring general practitioners to refer patients to them, by offering hefty commissions and various 'marketing' strategies. On the other hand, rational, ethical doctors working in smaller set-ups may not be able to attract many newer patients. Patients may be referred to specific hospitals by certain unscrupulous doctors who receive commissions, and patients themselves may also be drawn in by the ambience of 'five-star' hospitals. Thus, a negative spiral linked with gross commercialization has been set in motion today, and the situation is continually deteriorating. In this scenario, patients in search of rational, ethical doctors, and similarly, such doctors who would like to practise ethically, without giving commissions and cuts to ensure patients, are both in a bind.

A solution would be to replace the negative spiral with a positive spiral, which would benefit both patients and rational, ethical doctors.

The formation of 'Citizen–Doctor forums' in various cities and districts could promote such a positive spiral, by bridging the communication gap between these two sections that need each other. If such a forum is formed in each city/district, it would benefit both sections, and would also induce more doctors to step out of the commission-based rat race, and practise ethically. Some public-minded individuals or social groups need to engage with a few rational and ethical doctors in their area to initiate such a process. One essential ingredient for success would be the availability of at least a few rational and ethical doctors to start with, who would devote some time and energy for this activity. A second important component would be the presence of a committed social group or NGO, which may work as the secretariat of such a forum, particularly keeping in mind that most doctors are quite busy and may not be able to devote much time for coordination of such an activity.

The core activity of such a forum would naturally be informing patients about some appropriate, rational doctors, based on their specific conditions and requirements. As far as possible, the options of a few providers would be given, enabling the patient to make the actual choice based on their own specific requirements and preferences. Along with this, regular public discussions could be conducted to promote interaction between doctors and citizens on key issues like: What would be a desirable form of regulating private hospitals? What are patients' rights and responsibilities? What is a rational approach to common conditions like childbirth, or measures like child vaccination? The 'Citizen–Doctor forums' would need to be given wide publicity so that large numbers of citizens and more doctors would progressively join the group.

It must be underlined here, that at the time of initiating such a process in any area, clear criteria and procedures for including names of specific physicians in the list of rational and ethical doctors would have to be worked out. The forum could come out with a list of basic conditions that the involved doctors would need to sign, for being included in the list. This might include a poster display in the clinic on patients' rights, and a personal declaration that the doctor respects these rights; a declaration that the doctor does not take gifts and favours from pharmaceutical companies; a commitment to answering patients' queries and following rational treatment practices etc. At the same time, feedback from individual patients regarding each doctor would need to be analysed and taken into account, and if any doctor is found not following the basic criteria or declarations made by them, then they might be removed from the list. At the same time, doctors who have been positively rated by large numbers of patients would be appreciated and continued in the forum.

Some of the exchanges in the forum related to health awareness topics, rational treatment practices etc. could be mediated through a web portal or online platform. However, care would need to be taken that at no stage, or in any form, is an individual doctor or hospital allowed to advertise through this kind of a platform.

Provided that the forum gets strong support from a number of rational and ethical doctors, it can start something like a second opinion service, whereby patients could choose from among a panel of rational and ethical specialists, to seek a second opinion (some appropriate fee could be charged for providing such opinions). Based on the demands of the forum's work, a person could be assigned to respond to the queries coming from patients, and for coordinating activities.

Such Citizen–Doctor Forums are an emerging idea in the Indian setting. In this context, a notable voluntary service is currently run by the Hospital Guide Foundation, where referral advice is provided to patients free of charge in certain major cities.

Hospital Guide Foundation— Connecting Patients with Quality Health Care Providers

Hospital Guide Foundation (HGF)[1] is an NGO with a vision to revolutionize health care in India, by bridging gaps to make quality health care accessible across all sections of society. It is a free service that does not charge its patients, and also does not have any commercial transaction with suggested health care providers/doctors, hence ensuring unbiased suggestions. HGF's current core service, focused in Bangalore and Delhi, provides health care solutions by referring patients to appropriate doctors. HGF affiliates itself with practitioners after doing a reference check, so that the best of advice can be given to patients. HGF draws upon the goodwill and help of doctors both in private and government sectors. Every patient request is strongly evaluated and given equal importance, and then the patient is referred to the appropriate specialty/doctor. This methodology gives the patient a fair chance in getting the correct diagnosis, prognosis and treatment.

HGF also offers a platform via Facebook for doctors, hospitals, research scholars and the public to share experiences, ideas and opinions on subjects like generic drugs vs. branded drugs and other health care topics to raise public awareness.

Other such efforts are also emerging in the Indian context. These experiences need to be learned from, to help further generalize such forums.[2]

Contributing to the Health Movement, to Ensure Changes in the Health System

Active citizens, community organizations, consumer groups, social movements and progressive political representatives need to strengthen the movement for reforming the current unacceptable reality of the health sector. We should not forget that due to the vagaries of the human body, many of us may have to care for a patient among our family or friends in the coming period, and each of us could become a patient at some time during our lifetime. The situation now is frightening and is reaching a breaking point. We cannot afford to waste time; there is need for social action *now*.

Only if the demand for a rationalized, socially-regulated private medical sector becomes a public demand, will we be able to say that the doctors whose voices have been reflected in these pages have received constructive support from society. This needs to include a definite articulation of patients' rights, which have been outlined in the previous pages. And given the background that India is aspiring to become a global superpower, which can make a rocket reach the planet Mars, we also need to start asking whether our systems can also ensure that basic health care reaches every resident of the country. The approach of Universal Health Care, which could ensure good quality health care for all—free at the point of accessing care—now needs to be brought into social discourse and the political agenda.

We are hopeful that this can happen. Society will have to take many of the steps mentioned in the previous chapters to ensure social accountability of the private medical sector. This will not be an easy process; rather it may be a complex and contested process, since powerful commercial interests in the health sector might resist such changes. As part of this process, we will need to keep our eyes open and actively involve rational, ethical doctors as valuable allies to help in operationalizing rational treatment protocols, developing appropriate standards for hospitals, and drawing up charters of rights for patients as well as health care providers. We will need to support these doctors, while also seeking their support in such a larger movement.

Reflecting on 'Medical Consumerism'—Propagating Rational Health Practices

While reshaping the health care system is an important front of action, we also need to reshape social attitudes and conceptions regarding health and health care. Awareness campaigns are needed to convince people to avoid seeking irrational health care, and to promote healthy lifestyles as well as a rational approach to health care. Medical consumerism, irrational demand for unnecessary health care interventions (irrational injections, operations, investigations etc.) must be actively curbed through social action. A healthy society is not one which consumes more and more health care—rather it is one which needs less health care. Towards this goal, besides ensuring regulation and standard treatment guidelines to constrain irrational care in the private medical sector, there should be large-scale public education campaigns launched through the mass media; these topics should be made part of the school curriculum, and social movements should include these themes in their agenda.

And as citizens, we also need some introspection. Are we also becoming victims of medical consumerism by blindly believing that more health care and more expensive health care is always better? Aren't we on the wrong track if we think that by spending more money, consuming more medicines, undergoing operations and investigations at the drop of a hat, whether clearly indicated or not, we will be able to improve our health? We need to question some of these assumptions. Health care needs to be treated as a basic right and social good, not as a commodity. We will have to impress this upon ourselves, and also on the health care establishment and the government.

In Conclusion

The doctors whose voices of conscience are reflected in these pages have shown significant courage in moving beyond the denial mode one often finds among medical professionals, and have presented a grim yet realistic picture of the private medical sector in India today. We should appreciate that there are some such doctors active even now, who strive to practise medicine rationally and on the basis of professional ethics, despite myriad pressures and inducements to do otherwise. As we end this book, let us express our heartfelt gratitude to these doctors, and assure them that we will not let such doctors vanish; we will do whatever is possible to prevent them from becoming an extinct species.

Healing the health sector in India is going to be a long journey. As one step, those readers who are interested in knowing more, and getting involved can visit the websites *www.sathicehat. org* and *www.privatehospitalswatch.org.* We are confident that a process can be started whereby health and health services will become a right for everyone. Public health services can be made stronger, efficient and responsive, and this can be complemented by effectively regulating private health care providers. There will be guidelines regarding treatment and investigations, and doctors will be guided by these while carrying out treatment and investigations, minimizing irrational practices. As we move towards a UHC system, no one will have to pay for health care services at the time of service. Making sick people better will not be the only aim of health services; they will also actively work to prevent disease and promote good health. There will be adequate policy emphasis and expenditure on programmes that foster better health, including nutrition, clean water, sanitation and safe environments, which are today neglected as compared to curative services. Economic status, urban or rural location, gender, caste, religion or age would not prevent anyone from accessing quality health care.

This is not just a dream, this can become a reality, if people from various backgrounds and from different parts of the country join hands and start building a movement in this direction.

The patient is in critical condition. The time to start the treatment is now.

We thus find ourselves at a crossroads: health care can be considered a commodity to be sold, or it can be considered a basic social right.

It cannot comfortably be considered both of these at the same time.

This, I believe, is the great drama of medicine at the start of this century. And this is the choice before all people of faith and good will in these dangerous times.

—Dr Paul Farmer, *Pathologies of Power*[3]

An Appeal to Citizens

After reading this book, you might be feeling shocked, dismayed or concerned about the state of health care in the private sector in India. Maybe you already knew about these issues through your own experience, and this book may just confirm your understanding about what is going on in private hospitals. It is also possible that you may have positive experiences with certain individual doctors, who are trying to practise rationally and ethically despite the pressures of commercialization of health care.

In any of these situations, you may feel that something definitely needs to be done to change the situation, to ensure that all private hospitals respect patients' rights and provide rational and ethical care, with standardization of rates. At a broader level, you may also agree that major policy changes are needed to ensure that good quality, rational health care is made available to everyone as an entitlement. If you are thinking in this direction, then you would be glad to know that there are thousands of people in this country like yourself, who have a deep sense of concern around these issues in the health sector, and are trying to change this situation. In case you want to know more, and feel like contributing to ongoing efforts and campaigns around these issues, you can see the following websites and contact us on the email address given below:

www.privatehospitalswatch.org

www.sathicehat.org

www.phmindia.org

healthrightsindia@gmail.com

An Appeal to Doctors

If you are a practising doctor or have experience of medical practice in India, then the issues pointed out by various doctors speaking through the pages of this book would surely not be new to you. You might have some differences about the proposed 'treatments', but hopefully you would agree with the 'diagnosis' that the practices being adopted by many private hospitals today are a matter of concern, creating a dilemma among doctors who want to work in a principled and humane manner in the current situation. An individual doctor may try their best to practise rationally and ethically, but to do so and survive in the current competitive and commercialized environment, is not an easy proposition. Naturally, individual efforts are necessary but not sufficient to deal with this challenge, which require like-minded doctors to start interacting with each other, exploring ways to move beyond the current conundrum.

If you face such dilemmas and questions as a medical professional, then it would be clear from the voices of seventy-eight doctors reflected in this book, that you are not alone. A significant and growing number of doctors across India are now speaking up regarding the distortions and malpractices in the private medical sector. A national network has been initiated, involving doctors who are interested in promoting ethical, rational health care along with de-commercialization of the health sector. Meetings of such like-minded doctors are being organized in various cities and states across the country. If you would like to be part of these conversations and processes, then you can see the website and write to this email address:

www.ethicaldoctors.org
ethicaldoctorsindia@gmail.com

Endnotes

Introduction

1. *Rational health care* is based on standard approaches as described in medical textbooks and evidence-based guidelines, where ensuring optimal benefit to the patient is the sole consideration while recommending treatment. On the other hand, *irrational health care* is characterized by systematic deviation from such standard approaches and guidelines, which is often influenced by considerations of increasing the income of the hospital or doctor, rather than optimal benefit of the patient.
2. This is similar to the process of 'chain sampling' that is used to study individuals with rare traits, who may be easier to trace through informal contacts.

Chapter 1

1. Public hospitals in Mumbai.

Chapter 8

1. Charter of Patients' Rights and Responsibilities. JAA, Rugna Hakka Samiti, IMA, Pune.
2. Supreme Court Judgement, *Parmanand Katara v. Union of India* (1989).

3. Judgement of National Consumer Disputes Redressal Commission, *Pravat Kumar Mukherjee v. Ruby General Hospital & Others (2005).*

4. MCI Code of Ethics sections 2.1 and 2.4.

5. MCI Code of Ethics section 1.8 'Payment of Professional Services': A physician should announce his fees before rendering the service and not after the operation or treatment is under way. Remuneration received for such services should be in the form and amount specifically announced to the patient at the time the service is rendered.

6. Section 9(i), Clinical Establishments (Central Government) Rules, 2012.

7. MCI Code of Ethics section 1.3.2: If any request is made for medical records either by the patients/authorized attendant or legal authorities involved, the same may be duly acknowledged and documents shall be issued within the period of 72 hours.

8. Central Information Commission Judgement, *Nisha Priya Bhatia* v. *Institute of HB&AS*, GNCTD (2014).

9. Charter of Patients' Rights and Responsibilities. JAA, Rugna Hakka Samiti, IMA, Pune.

10. See an analysis of the views of twenty-eight physicians, ethicists and sociologists on the second opinion in: Pandya, Sunil. 'Some opinions on the second opinion'. *Indian Journal of Medical Ethics*, 6:1, 1998.

11. MCI Code of Ethics sections 2.2, 7.14 and 7.17.

12. MCI Code of Ethics section 7.16.

13. Judgement of National Consumer Disputes Redressal Commission, *Meenu Jain & Prem Chand Jain v. Fortis Health Management (North) Ltd (2013).*

14. MCI Code of Ethics section 1.5.

15. 'Ethical concerns in clinical trials in India: an investigation by Sandhya Srinivasan'. Centre for Study of Ethics and Rights, Mumbai, 2009.

16. 'Exploratory Study on Clinical Trials Conducted by Swiss Pharmaceutical Companies in India: Issues, Concerns and

Challenges'. *Berne Declaration*, SAMA (ed.), Lausanne/Zurich/ New Delhi, 2013.

17. Pulikuthiyil, George et al. 'Regulation of Drug and Clinical Trials in India: Why RIGHTS Matter'. *Jananeethi*, 2011.

18. See www.unethicalclinicaltrial.org.

19. 'Ethical Guidelines for Biomedical Research on Human Participants'. Indian Council of Medical Research, New Delhi, 2006.

20. 'World Medical Assembly Declaration of Helsinki: Ethical Principles for Medical Research Involving Human Subjects', available at *www.wma.net/en/30publications/10policies/b3/17c.pdf.*

21. Sequeira, Rosy. 'Detaining patients over unpaid bills is "inhuman", Bombay High Court says'. *Times of India*, 13 June 2014.

22. *Times of India*, Mumbai, 1 July 2014.

23. Madhani, Apurva. 'Bombay High Court laments over commercialization of health services; slams City-Hospital for detaining patient over disputed bills'. *LiveLaw.in*, 13 June 2014.

24. This section is adapted from information available on the website of ACASH (Association for Consumers' Action on Safety and Health): www.acash.org/newsletter1.htm.

25. Shenoy, P. D. *Medical Negligence: What Doctors, Patients & Hospitals Should Know.* Sterling Publishers, 2013.

26. Koley, T.K. *Medical Negligence and the Law in India: Duties, Responsibilities, Rights.* Oxford University Press, 2013.

27. Joga Rao, S.V. 'Medical negligence liability under the consumer protection act: A review of judicial perspective'. *Indian J Urol.* July–September, 25:3, pp. 361–371. 2009.

28. Murthy, K.K.S.R. 'Medical negligence and the law'. *Indian Journal of Medical Ethics*, 4:3. 2007.

Chapter 9

1. The major ideas in this section draw upon a useful piece on 'Good Medical Practice' by Peter Rubin, given on the website of the General Medical Council of UK: www.gmc-uk.org/guidance/10058.asp.

2. Emanuel, E.J. and L.L. Emanuel. 'Four Models of the physician–patient relationship'. *Journal of American Medical Association*, 267: 16. 1992.

Chapter 10

1. This section and the next section is partly based on a portion of the paper: Phadke, A., More, A., Shukla, A., and A. Gadre. 'Developing an approach towards social accountability of private health care services'. SATHI, India and COPASAH, 2013.
2. Brazil has developed a 'Unified Health System' which includes public health services as well as a section of private hospitals under a publicly organized and funded system. The health councils are participatory bodies which plan and monitor services by both public and private providers, who are part of the Unified Health System. This is one of the few large-scale models of participatory oversight of public as well as contracted private providers. For further details see Phadke et al, 2013.

Chapter 11

1. This chapter is an adapted, shortened and updated version of the booklet 'Twenty Questions and Answers about a System for Universal Health Care', published by SATHI in 2012. The primary drafting of this booklet was done by Dr Amita Pitre, with editing by Dr Anant Phadke.
2. The terms Universal Health Care and Universal Health Coverage are often used interchangeably. But it should be noted that from the point of view of many public health experts and health activists, these two terms do not have the same implications. It is not merely a question of extending 'coverage' by the existing form of health care provisioning, but of transforming it to a new system, which can ensure availability of health care as a right and not as a commodity. Hence, here we have used the concept and term: 'Universal Health Care'.

3. This section draws upon a set of principles that were suggested by certain members of Medico Friends Circle to the High Level Expert Group on UHC. Many of these principles are reflected in the HLEG report.

4. See the film 'Sicko' by Michael Moore to understand the serious problems that people currently face related to inadequate health care protection in the US.

5. See www.cbmpmaharashtra.org.

6. See www.nrhmcommunityaction.org.

Chapter 12

1. The Hospital Guide Foundation (HGF) was co-founded by Indiritta Singh D'mello and Manu Tripathi in 2010. For more information, see www.hospitalguide.in.

2. Farmer, Paul. *Pathologies of Power*. University of California Press, 2004.

Index

A Note on the Authors

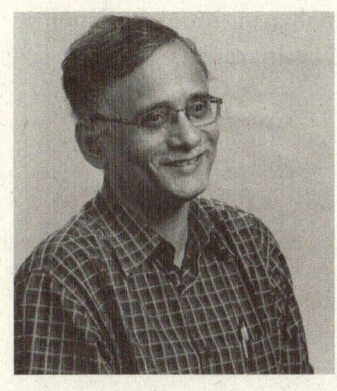

Dr Arun Gadre is a gynaecologist. He practised in a drought-prone area of rural Maharashtra for twenty years. With the support of his anaesthetist wife, Dr Jyoti Gadre, he ran a small private hospital, witnessing first-hand the degeneration of the once noble medical profession. Unable to stem the rot and fatigued by practising in a resource-poor set-up with rising patient expectations, he left private practice to work as a coordinator of a Pune-based NGO, SATHI, which specializes in policy advocacy related to health care in India. Dr Gadre is the author of seventeen books in Marathi, including six novels, and has received several literary awards.

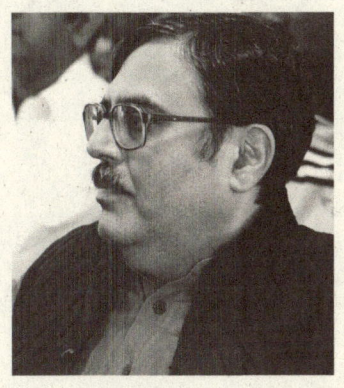

Dr Abhay Shukla is a public health physician, with a postgraduate degree in community medicine from the All India Institute of Medical Sciences, New Delhi. He

189

has worked on health issues in collaboration with people's movements and grassroots NGOs in Maharashtra for two decades. He is a senior programme coordinator with SATHI, Pune, and is a member of advisory bodies for the National Rural Health Mission and the National Human Rights Commission. He is a national convener of Jan Swasthya Abhiyan (People's Health Movement–India) and has facilitated public hearings on the right to health care across the country. Dr Shukla has authored and edited several books on health system issues. He has contributed to developing the framework of community-based monitoring and planning of health services at the national level and in Maharashtra. He is involved in action and research for the promotion of patients' rights, the social regulation of the private medical sector and universal health care.